Traumatic Dental Injuries in Children

Rebecca L. Slayton · Elizabeth A. Palmer

Traumatic Dental Injuries in Children

A Clinical Guide to Management and Prevention

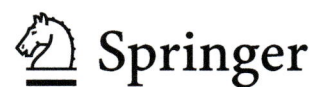 Springer

Rebecca L. Slayton
Department of Pediatric Dentistry
University of Washington School
of Dentistry
Seattle, WA
USA

Elizabeth A. Palmer
Department of Pediatric Dentistry
Oregon Health & Science University School
of Dentistry
Portland, OR
USA

ISBN 978-3-030-25795-8   ISBN 978-3-030-25793-4   (eBook)
https://doi.org/10.1007/978-3-030-25793-4

This Springer imprint is published by the registered company Springer Nature Switzerland AG
The registered company address is: Gewerbestrasse 11, 6330 Cham, Switzerland

Preface

Traumatic injuries that involve the teeth and mouth are common and frequently devastating for the individual involved. Strategies to prevent or minimize the risk of traumatic dental injuries in children should be a part of the anticipatory guidance that all dentists provide to their patients and families.

This book is meant to be a clinical guide for dentists, educators, and dental students to increase awareness of ways to prevent and manage traumatic dental injuries in children. The challenges that are unique to young children and children with special health care needs are discussed and techniques for addressing these needs are described.

Because traumatic injuries occur unexpectedly, dental and other health care providers need to have an easily accessible resource available to them to ensure timely and appropriate treatment is provided. This book is intended to serve as that resource and to complement the existing trauma guidelines developed by the International Association of Dental Traumatology.

Seattle, WA, USA   Rebecca L. Slayton
Portland, OR, USA   Elizabeth A. Palmer

Contents

1 Introduction: Epidemiology of Traumatic Dental Injuries 1
  1.1 Pediatric Trauma 1
  1.2 Trauma Management Education 2
  1.3 Incidence of TDIs. 3
    1.3.1 Birth to 5 Years. 3
    1.3.2 Age 6–12 Years 4
    1.3.3 Age 13–18 years 4
  1.4 Risk Factors 5
    1.4.1 Sports 5
    1.4.2 Overjet 5
    1.4.3 Bicycles 6
    1.4.4 Automobile 6
    1.4.5 Violence 6
    1.4.6 Attention-Deficit/Hyperactivity Disorder (ADHD). 7
    1.4.7 Tongue Piercing. 8
    1.4.8 Chronic Health Conditions or Physical Limitations 9
    1.4.9 Iatrogenic Injuries 10
  1.5 Treatment and Timing 11
  1.6 Guidelines 12
  References. 12

2 Unique Challenges in the Pediatric Population 17
  2.1 Behavior Guidance. 17
  2.2 Behavior Guidance Considerations 18
    2.2.1 Tell-Show-Do. 19
    2.2.2 Positive Reinforcement 19
    2.2.3 Distraction 19
    2.2.4 Voice Control 20
    2.2.5 Escape 20
    2.2.6 Parent Presence 20
    2.2.7 Deferred Treatment 21
    2.2.8 Nitrous Oxide. 21
  2.3 Advanced Behavior Guidance Techniques 22
    2.3.1 Protective Stabilization 22

		2.3.2	Minimal Sedation	24
		2.3.3	Moderate Sedation	25
		2.3.4	General Anesthesia	25
	2.4	Consent		25
	2.5	Communication		26
	2.6	Parental Presence		26
	2.7	Growth and Development Considerations		27
	2.8	Child Abuse		27
	References			28
3	**Physical Examination and Diagnosis**			31
	3.1	Initial Assessment		31
	3.2	Patient/Family Interview		33
	3.3	Medical History		33
	3.4	Neurologic Evaluation		34
	3.5	Extraoral/Intraoral Examination		35
		3.5.1	Extraoral Examination	36
		3.5.2	Intraoral Examination	36
	3.6	Radiographic Evaluation		37
	3.7	Dental Office Preparation		39
	References			40
4	**Primary Tooth Crown and Root Fractures**			43
	4.1	Uncomplicated Crown Fracture		43
		4.1.1	Treatment Recommendations	44
		4.1.2	Prognosis	46
		4.1.3	Sequelae	46
		4.1.4	Behavior Management	46
	4.2	Complicated Crown Fracture		47
		4.2.1	Treatment Recommendations	47
		4.2.2	Follow-Up	48
		4.2.3	Prognosis	48
		4.2.4	Sequelae	49
		4.2.5	Behavior Management	49
	4.3	Crown/Root Fracture		50
		4.3.1	Treatment Recommendations	50
		4.3.2	Follow-Up	51
		4.3.3	Prognosis	51
		4.3.4	Sequelae	52
		4.3.5	Behavior Management	52
	4.4	Root Fracture		52
		4.4.1	Treatment Recommendations	53
		4.4.2	Follow-Up	54
		4.4.3	Prognosis	54
		4.4.4	Sequelae	54
		4.4.5	Behavior Management	54

	4.5	Fractures of the Alveolar Process.	55
		4.5.1 Treatment Recommendations	55
		4.5.2 Follow-Up	56
		4.5.3 Prognosis	56
		4.5.4 Sequelae	56
		4.5.5 Behavior Management	56
	4.6	Patient Instructions.	56
		References.	57
5	**Primary Tooth Luxation Injuries**		**59**
	5.1	Concussion and Subluxation	59
		5.1.1 Treatment Recommendations	59
		5.1.2 Follow-Up	60
		5.1.3 Prognosis	60
		5.1.4 Sequelae	61
		5.1.5 Behavior Guidance.	61
	5.2	Lateral Luxation.	61
		5.2.1 Treatment Recommendations	62
		5.2.2 Follow-Up	63
		5.2.3 Prognosis	63
		5.2.4 Sequelae	64
		5.2.5 Behavior Guidance.	64
	5.3	Extrusive Luxation.	64
		5.3.1 Treatment Recommendations	65
		5.3.2 Follow-Up	65
		5.3.3 Prognosis	65
		5.3.4 Sequelae	66
		5.3.5 Behavior Guidance.	66
	5.4	Intrusive Luxation	67
		5.4.1 Treatment Recommendations	68
		5.4.2 Follow-Up	69
		5.4.3 Prognosis	69
		5.4.4 Sequelae	70
		5.4.5 Behavior Guidance.	70
	5.5	Avulsion.	70
		5.5.1 Treatment.	71
		5.5.2 Follow-Up	71
		5.5.3 Prognosis	71
		5.5.4 Sequelae	72
		5.5.5 Tooth Replacement Options.	72
	5.6	Patient Instructions.	74
		References.	75
6	**Permanent Tooth Crown and Root Fractures**		**77**
	6.1	Clinical and Radiographic Examination	77
	6.2	Uncomplicated Crown Fracture.	78

      6.2.1   Enamel Fracture 78

      6.2.2   Enamel and Dentin Fracture 79

  6.3   Complicated Crown Fracture 84

      6.3.1   Treatment Recommendations 86

      6.3.2   Follow-Up 92

      6.3.3   Prognosis 92

      6.3.4   Sequelae 93

  6.4   Crown-Root Fracture: Uncomplicated 93

      6.4.1   Treatment Recommendations 94

      6.4.2   Follow-Up 97

      6.4.3   Prognosis 97

  6.5   Crown/Root Fracture: Complicated 97

      6.5.1   Treatment Recommendations 97

      6.5.2   Follow-Up 103

      6.5.3   Prognosis 103

  6.6   Root Fracture 103

      6.6.1   Treatment Recommendations 104

      6.6.2   Follow-Up 106

      6.6.3   Prognosis 106

  6.7   Alveolar Fracture 106

      6.7.1   Treatment Recommendations 107

      6.7.2   Follow-Up 107

      6.7.3   Prognosis 107

  References 108

7 Permanent Tooth Luxation Injuries 111

  7.1   Concussion 111

      7.1.1   Treatment Recommendations 111

      7.1.2   Follow-Up 112

      7.1.3   Prognosis 112

  7.2   Subluxation 112

      7.2.1   Treatment Recommendations 113

      7.2.2   Follow-Up 113

      7.2.3   Prognosis 113

  7.3   Lateral Luxation 114

      7.3.1   Treatment Recommendations 116

      7.3.2   Follow-Up 116

      7.3.3   Prognosis 117

  7.4   Extrusive Luxation 118

      7.4.1   Treatment Recommendations 119

      7.4.2   Follow-Up 119

      7.4.3   Prognosis 119

  7.5   Intrusion 120

      7.5.1   Treatment Recommendations 121

      7.5.2   Follow-Up 122

7.5.3 Prognosis 124
References. 125

8 Permanent Tooth Avulsion Injuries 127
8.1 Pulpal Reactions. 129
8.2 Periodontal Reactions 129
8.3 Treatment Guidelines. 130
8.4 Triage Protocol. 131
8.5 Transport/Storage Media 133
8.6 Immature Teeth Replanted Immediately or Within 60 min 134
8.6.1 Treatment Recommendations 134
8.6.2 Follow-Up 137
8.6.3 Prognosis 137
8.7 Immature Teeth with Extraoral Dry Time Greater Than 60 min 138
8.7.1 Treatment Recommendations 138
8.7.2 Follow-Up 139
8.7.3 Prognosis 139
8.8 Mature Teeth Replanted Immediately or Within 60 min 139
8.8.1 Treatment Recommendations 139
8.8.2 Follow-Up 141
8.8.3 Prognosis 143
8.9 Mature Teeth with Extraoral Dry Time Greater Than 60 min 143
8.9.1 Treatment Recommendations 143
8.9.2 Follow-Up 144
8.9.3 Prognosis 144
References. 144

9 Sequelae and Management Options 147
9.1 Tooth Discoloration 147
9.2 Pulpal Necrosis 148
9.2.1 Treatment of a Nonvital Primary Tooth 148
9.2.2 Treatment of a Nonvital Immature Permanent Tooth 149
9.2.3 Treatment of a Nonvital Mature Permanent Tooth 150
9.3 Pulp Canal Obliteration 150
9.4 Inflammatory Resorption 151
9.4.1 Internal Inflammatory Resorption 151
9.4.2 External Inflammatory Resorption. 152
9.4.3 Treatment Recommendations 153
9.5 Ankylosis/Replacement Resorption. 153
9.5.1 Treatment of Ankylosed Primary Teeth 154
9.5.2 Treatment of Ankylosed Permanent Teeth. 154
9.6 Premature Loss of Primary Tooth 156
9.7 Damage to the Succedaneous Tooth by the Injured Primary Tooth. . 157
9.7.1 Enamel Defects 157
9.7.2 Crown and Root Dilaceration 158
9.7.3 Altered Eruption Timing or Direction 160

9.8 Permanent Tooth Replacement Options in the Growing Child 160
    9.8.1 Temporary Partial Dentures 160
    9.8.2 Autotransplantation 161
References 161

10 Prevention of Traumatic Dental Injuries 167
  10.1 Child-Proofing Homes 167
  10.2 Sports: Helmets/Mouthguards 168
    10.2.1 Mouthguard Types and Fabrication 169
  10.3 Bicycle: Helmets 172
  10.4 Excessive Overjet 173
  10.5 Attention-Deficit Hyperactivity Disorder (ADHD) 173
  10.6 Automobile Injuries 174
  10.7 Violence 174
  10.8 Summary 176
References 176

Introduction: Epidemiology of Traumatic Dental Injuries

Traumatic dental injuries (TDIs) occur at all ages and although there are ways to limit these injuries, they are not completely preventable. The etiology is complex and includes oral characteristics of the individual such as excessive overjet, factors related to human behavior such as risk-taking or impulsiveness and environmental factors including socioeconomic status and/or deprivation [1]. Within the behavioral component, the etiology can be further divided into intentional and unintentional causes, where unintentional refers to falls or collisions and intentional is more likely to involve a violent act that is either self or other inflicted [1]. It is thought that violent injuries may be under reported because often when the injury was reported, the intent was not divulged.

1.1 Pediatric Trauma

Unintentional injuries vary with age. Toddlers fall as they are learning to walk. School-aged children fall during play or sustain injuries during sporting activities. Adolescents and adults may get injured while participating in sports, on bicycles or in cars. Children with special health care needs (SHCN) often have poor coordination or limited mobility. The risk for injury is always there. In a review of the literature in 2008, Glendor reported that one-third of all children had sustained a TDI to primary dentition and one-fourth of all school-aged children had experienced a TDI to the permanent dentition [1]. Recently, Petti and colleagues investigated the incidence and prevalence of TDIs worldwide [2]. They reported the world prevalence of TDIs to primary teeth to be 21% and for permanent teeth, 15%. Their study demonstrated that TDIs are the second most frequent oral disease with dental caries being the most frequent. A recent systematic review and meta-analysis of the prevalence and etiology of TDIs in children evaluated 44 papers from countries throughout the world [3]. These authors estimated the prevalence of dental trauma in children and adolescents to be 17.5%. Injuries were more common in boys. The most common

© Springer Nature Switzerland AG 2020
R. L. Slayton, E. A. Palmer, *Traumatic Dental Injuries in Children*,
https://doi.org/10.1007/978-3-030-25793-4_1

cause of dental trauma was from falls at home with enamel fracture being the more frequent type of injury [3].

TDIs in children present challenges beyond what is experienced in more mature patients. In very young children, a traumatic dental injury may be the reason for their first visit to the dentist. This adds to an already potentially emotionally charged visit for both the child and the parent or caregiver. In this situation, the dentist has not had the opportunity to establish rapport or instill confidence and trust in their abilities to provide appropriate care for the child. Even if this is not the child's first dental visit, traumatic injuries and the treatment required are often beyond the ability of the child to tolerate. Pediatric dentists are skilled in behavior guidance techniques. However, many of the more advanced techniques such as sedation and general anesthesia require advanced planning and may not be available for emergencies in the office.

Fearful or anxious patients of any age present additional challenges and these behavioral challenges must be taken into account at the time of the initial assessment and treatment plan. Proper management of most TDIs requires multiple visits to the dental office over a period of months or years. Children or adolescents who are unable to comply with recommended treatment may require modifications to what is considered "ideal." In addition, these modifications may adversely affect the prognosis of the injured tooth and should be carefully explained to the caregiver and patient.

Children with SHCN and/or complex medical diagnoses may also present behavioral challenges due to their inability to understand or cooperate for treatment in the traditional dental setting.

This book will focus on the unique characteristics of children and adolescents that significantly influence how TDIs are managed. Because the person responsible for a child's well-being may be a parent, foster parent, grandparent, or other relative, throughout this book, the adult who is responsible for a child or adolescent patient will be referred to as caregiver.

1.2   Trauma Management Education

Considering how frequently dental injuries occur, it is unfortunate how little time is spent in the dental school curriculum regarding prevention and treatment of dental traumatic injuries. The Commission on Dental Accreditation Standards for Dental Education Programs state that "graduates must be competent in providing oral health care within the scope of general dentistry, as defined by the school, including: dental emergencies." This leaves a lot of room for interpretation of what is meant by "dental emergencies." Management of TDIs may be discussed in courses offered by the pediatric dentistry, endodontics, and oral surgery departments, but the depth of information provided varies considerably. In the standards for advanced education in pediatric dentistry, in-depth didactic education in the "care of orofacial injuries in infants, children, and adolescents" as well as clinical competence in managing these injuries is expected [4]. The standards are similar for Advanced Specialty Education

Programs in Endodontics with the stated intent: "To ensure that students/residents are trained to manage all aspects of the endodontic care of teeth with traumatic injuries" [5].

Studies regarding the proper management of TDIs in the primary and permanent dentition have shown a general lack of knowledge among dentists worldwide. Ravikumar et al. [6] surveyed general dentists regarding the management of injuries in the primary dentition. The authors reported that about half of the dentists responded accurately regarding the management of avulsed primary teeth, 55% answered appropriately for the management of luxated teeth and 36% for crown/root fractures.

The International Association of Dental Traumatology developed guidelines for the management of TDIs in 2001. They have been updated twice and are freely available to practicing dentists worldwide. In two recent studies, Hartmann et al. [7] and Alyasi et al. [8] surveyed practicing dentists to determine their knowledge of these guidelines. Hartmann and colleagues sent 14,753 surveys to registered dentists in Rio Grande do Sul. The response rate was low (9.59%) with only 1414 dentists participating. The authors judged the overall knowledge of the guidelines to be moderate with slightly higher knowledge for specialists in endodontics and pediatric dentistry [7]. Alyasi et al. compared knowledge of the trauma guidelines between general dentists and pediatric dentists in the United Arab Emirates. On average, general dentists correctly answered 37.5% of the questions and pediatric dentists answered 42.8% correctly. Both scores were considered a reflection of poor knowledge [8].

There is clearly a need for more education about management of TDIs for both general dentists and specialists.

1.3 Incidence of TDIs

There are significant differences in the cause of TDIs for different age groups. This is not surprising due to the types of behaviors that are most common for different ages. It is important to be aware of activities that put children at risk for dental injuries so that health care providers can educate families about ways to prevent or minimize injuries. This education is part of the anticipatory guidance that is provided during routine dental and medical visits.

1.3.1 Birth to 5 Years

From birth to 5 years of age, children are learning to walk, run, and climb. They are still developing coordination and may react impulsively. Dental trauma is most likely the result of a fall during this age group. One prospective study found that 25% of the children studied had a traumatic injury prior to their fourth birthday. The majority of injuries occurred inside the home and as the result of a fall [9]. The most common age for injuries in toddlers is between 18 and 30 months, reflecting the age that most children learn to walk [10].

Health care providers who treat children are mandated to recognize and report suspected child abuse. When the description of an injury provided by the caregiver does not match what is seen clinically, further investigation is warranted. More than half of child abuse cases involve craniofacial, head, face and neck injuries including fractured, displaced or avulsed teeth, and intraoral lacerations [11]. Careful assessment and investigation into the cause of the injury is imperative. When child abuse is suspected, the dentist must report their findings to the appropriate authorities in their state or country.

1.3.2   Age 6–12 Years

During the ages of 6–12 years, children are in school and spending most of the day out of the home. They participate in recess during school hours and may be involved in sports. The peak incidence for TDIs in this group has been reported to be between 9 and 10 years of age and the most common injury is an uncomplicated crown fracture [10]. The currently accepted terminology for fractures of teeth uses "uncomplicated" to describe fractures of enamel and/or dentin that do not involve a pulp exposure. Fractures that include a pulp exposure are called "complicated."

Among fifth and sixth grade children in Jerusalem, the most commonly traumatized teeth are maxillary incisors [12]. This is consistent with other studies that demonstrate that maxillary incisor trauma is correlated with the extent of incisor overjet [13]. For example, in a meta-analysis of traumatic injuries to incisors, 9% of the moderate to severe injuries occurred in individuals with less than 3 mm overjet while 32% occurred in those with greater than 6 mm overjet [13].

Recently, it was recognized that children and adolescents with Attention-Deficit/Hyperactivity Disorder (ADHD) are at increased risk for TDIs. When children with or without TDIs were evaluated for hyperactivity, those with higher hyperactivity scores were significantly more likely to have suffered a TDI [14]. Similarly, a review of 10 years of trauma literature concluded that ADHD is a significant risk factor for TDIs [15].

Children with SHCN are also at increased risk for dental trauma due to a number of factors including intellectual, behavioral, neurologic, and physical challenges [16]. In a cohort of school-aged children, 9% of the children with SHCN had experienced trauma compared to 4% of typically developed children [16].

1.3.3   Age 13–18 years

In children between the ages of 13 and 18 years, many of the same risk factors as those in the 6–12-year age group apply. However, in this age group, there are likely to be more contact sports and more time spent away from home for social and sporting activities. By age 13, individuals usually have complete permanent dentition and the consequences of serious dental trauma are long lasting. Adolescents often have the feeling of omnipotence and immortality, leading to risk-taking behavior, lack of impulse control, testing authority, and a shift away from dependence on caregivers.

1.4 Risk Factors

There are many activities, behaviors, and physical characteristics that put a child at increased risk for TDIs. Knowing what the risks are at the individual level provides an opportunity to develop a preventive plan for each patient that can be shared with caregivers. The more common risks for TDIs are discussed below. Preventive strategies are discussed in Chap. 10.

1.4.1 Sports

Most sports put children and adolescents at increased risk for traumatic injuries, including dental trauma. Protective equipment is recommended but not always enforced. In the United States, the National College Athletic Association (NCAA) and High School Athletic Association require the use of mouthguards for football, field hockey, ice hockey, and wrestling [17]. In spite of this, a study of sports injuries showed that in 72% of dental traumatic injuries, no mouthguard was worn [17].

1.4.2 Overjet

Maxillary central incisors are the most frequently traumatized teeth, followed by maxillary lateral incisors and mandibular incisors [18]. The susceptibility of maxillary incisors is increased by their extent of overjet (Fig. 1.1). In a meta-analysis of studies done over a 25-year period, having a large overjet doubled or tripled the risk for anterior tooth trauma [13]. In most studies, 6 mm is used as the threshold for large overjet. Even an overjet greater than 3 mm increases the risk for maxillary incisor trauma significantly.

Cavalleri et al. found that 40% of fractures to permanent teeth occurred in children with maxillary overjets greater than 3 mm [19].

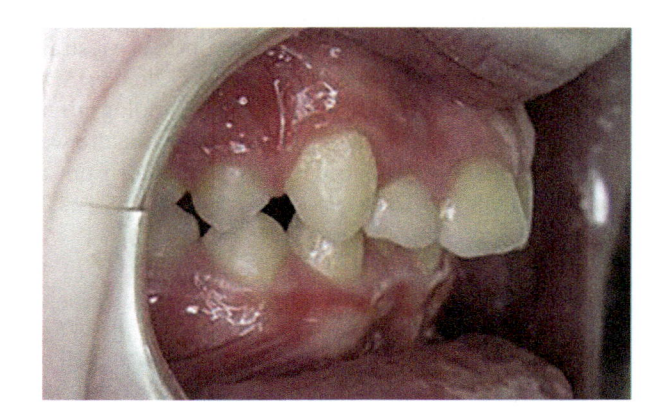

Fig. 1.1 In both the primary and permanent dentition, excess overjet increases the risk for traumatic dental injuries and maxillary incisors are the most frequently traumatized teeth

Borzabadi-Farahani et al. found that those most likely to have maxillary incisor trauma were boys, with class II sagittal skeletal relationship, and a decreased Frankfort-Mandibular Plane Angle (a short facial profile), and an overjet greater than 3.5 mm [20].

1.4.3 Bicycles

Accidents involving riding bicycles are relatively common and result in injuries to the head, limbs, and teeth. Twenty-two U.S. states require children to wear a bicycle helmet [21]. The age requirement varies by state and it is unclear how frequently these laws are enforced. Internationally, a number of countries have mandatory helmet laws either for all ages or just for children [21]. When worn properly, helmets protect against head injuries but may or may not protect against facial or dental injuries. Bicycle helmets have been shown to reduce both the number and severity of head injuries [22]. In addition, helmets have been shown to reduce the severity of upper and midface injuries but not lower face injuries [23]. Since the maxillary incisors are the teeth most frequently injured during falls, the use of a bicycle helmet should be encouraged to prevent both head injuries and dental injuries.

1.4.4 Automobile

Seat belts, car seats, and air bags have significantly decreased the number and severity of injuries related to automobile accidents. In the United States, the National Highway Traffic Safety Administration estimated that the use of seatbelts and airbags was 75% effective in preventing serious head injuries [24]. More recent data showed that seat belt use increased from 82.5% in 2007 to 90.1% in 2016 [25].

The incidence and severity of maxillofacial injuries occurred in 1 out of 449 accidents when the driver and passenger used both seat belts and airbags while this rate was 1 in 40 for individuals that used neither seat belts nor airbags [26]. Many states have laws regarding the use of child restraints such as car seats and booster seats. The lowest risk of injury occurs when age appropriate safety restraints are used in the rear seat of the car. Inappropriately restrained children were at almost twice the risk of injury and unrestrained children were at greater than three times the risk of injury [27]. A study focusing on the etiology of mandibular fractures reported that the most common cause of mandibular fracture was from road traffic accidents (68%) and the second most common was fall from a height (30%) [28]. In this study, the male to female ratio was 4.5:1.

1.4.5 Violence

Child maltreatment is a global issue that occurs at all ages. According to the World Health Organization, one-fourth of all adults report having been physically abused as children [29]. Although there have been a number of national surveys on this topic, the data from many countries is missing or incomplete. The Centers for Disease Control and Prevention provides access to data from Violence against Children Surveys (VACS) from a few countries [30]. These surveys report on incidence of physical and sexual abuse toward children under 18 years of age. Unfortunately, these surveys do not report data on dental or maxillofacial trauma.

In the United States, the most common age for physical maltreatment is in children under 7 years. National statistics in the U.S. demonstrate that of the children who died from child abuse, 70% were under 3 years of age [31].

Dentists are vital for the recognition and reporting of child abuse because they see children on a regular basis and because more than half of child abuse cases involve injuries to the head, face, and neck [11]. When the description of an injury does not match what is seen clinically, there should be further investigation. For example, preambulatory children rarely have bruises and bruises to the torso, ears, and neck in children under 4 are suggestive of abuse [32].

Fighting has been documented as one of the causes of dental trauma in adolescents. Maxillofacial trauma as a result of interpersonal violence (IPV) has been reported to have a prevalence rate ranging from 9 to 52% [33]. In a study of 790 patients with maxillofacial trauma from IPV, 17% were found to have dental trauma. These numbers included both domestic and urban violence. Four percent of those with dental trauma were under 19 years of age [33].

In a study of 6000 patients (of all ages) with facial injuries, 48% had dental trauma. Of those with dental trauma, 36% were from acts of violence [34].

One of the challenges of gathering reliable data about the prevalence of maxillofacial and dental trauma is that there is not a central repository for this information. For injuries that are primarily dental in nature, the patient is most likely seen by their dentist of record. If the injury is more extensive or involves the face, jaws, or head, the patient is more likely to be seen in a hospital emergency room and managed by a maxillofacial surgeon. National trauma databases exist in a number of countries and generally collect data for traumatic injuries requiring a visit to the emergency room or hospitalization. Some of these databases include maxillofacial injuries [35, 36] but not specifically TDIs.

In a study in the UK, 71% of maxillofacial injuries were due to a combination of assaults and traffic accidents [37].

1.4.6   Attention-Deficit/Hyperactivity Disorder (ADHD)

According to the ADHD Institute [38], the prevalence worldwide of this disorder for children and adolescents is between 5.3 and 7.1% making it one of the most common neurodevelopmental disorders of childhood. It affects individuals of all ages and has been reported to have a higher prevalence among males. The primary characteristics of ADHD are hyperactivity, inattentiveness and impulsivity. In addition, their increased accident proneness contributes to the risk for injury of all types, including dental [39].

It has been recognized for over 10 years that children and adolescents with ADHD are at increased risk for TDIs. In a recent review of the literature, 9 out of 12 studies confirmed the link between ADHD and TDI in children and adolescents [15]. The increased risk for dental trauma among children with ADHD is estimated to be three times that of children without ADHD [40].

1.4.7   Tongue Piercing

Tongue piercing has become more popular in the last decade or two and consists of one or more metal studs that extend from the dorsal to the ventral surface of the tongue and have balls screwed onto each end (Fig. 1.2). Numerous case reports have documented traumatic injuries to teeth caused by the tongue stud. The most common dental injuries are chipping or fracture of teeth and restorations, abrasion, and pulp injury [1].

Fig. 1.2 A double barbell type piercing shown from the (**a**) ventral and (**b**) dorsal surfaces of the tongue increases the risk for dental trauma. The habit of tapping them against the teeth or inadvertently biting down on the metal balls may cause traumatic dental injuries

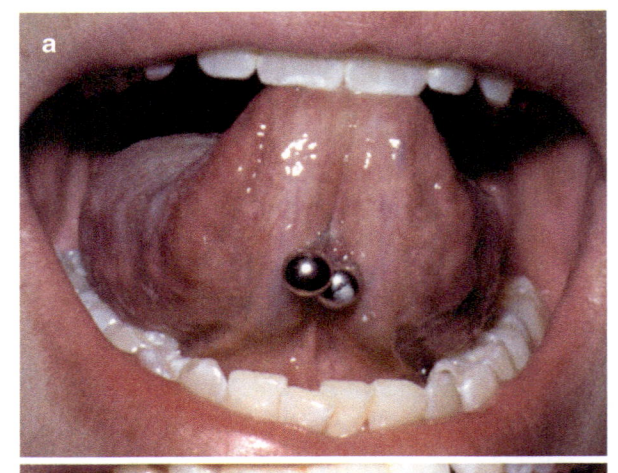

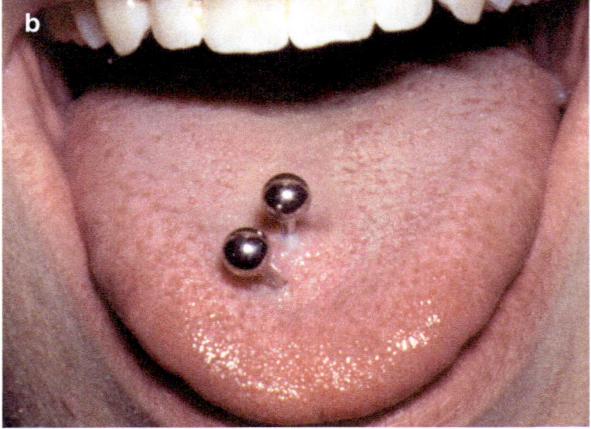

In a survey of University students, Mayers and Chiffriller [41], reported that 51% had body piercing. The medical complications associated with piercing had an incidence of 19%. Approximately 9% of the piercings were of the tongue. The most common piercing was the navel for women and the ear for men. In another study, Campbell et al. [42] evaluated the duration of piercing and its effect on lingual gingival recession and tooth chipping. Both findings increased with length of time worn. Lingual recession was most likely to occur in mandibular incisors and was evident in 19.2% of individuals after 2 years of wearing the stud. Molars and premolars were the most likely teeth to be chipped and this was more often seen after 4 years of wear. The prevalence of tooth chipping was also 19.2% but there was minimal overlap between those with recession and those with chipping [42].

Oral piercing is more common in older adolescents. Most states in the U.S. have regulations regarding body piercing. In 38 states there are laws that prohibit body piercing on minors without caregiver permission. Dentists who treat adolescents should be aware of the potential complications related to oral piercing and advise their patients about the risks.

1.4.8 Chronic Health Conditions or Physical Limitations

1.4.8.1 Epilepsy

Individuals with epilepsy are at increased risk for injury that is frequently seizure related. In a study of institutionalized patients with epilepsy, Besserman [43] reported that 52% had experienced one or more TDIs. One-third of these injuries were directly related to a fall during a seizure. In a study of children with epilepsy in Nigeria, 45.6% of the children with epilepsy reported having experienced seizure-related injuries in the past year compared to 20.8% of the children in the control group [44]. Of the children with seizure-related injuries, 43% involved the tongue, mouth, head, or teeth and 8% involved injury to teeth that resulted in tooth loss.

1.4.8.2 Cerebral Palsy

Cerebral palsy (CP) is a condition with central motor deficit that is often initiated prenatally or perinatally. In some cases, it can be the result of a hypoxic event in childhood. It often results in a child relying on a wheel chair or other forms of assistance for mobility. They may also have difficulty controlling involuntary movements. Because of these characteristics, they are more prone to falls than children without CP. There have been a number of studies focused on dental traumatic injuries for children with SHCN and developmental disabilities, including cerebral palsy.

Al-Batayneh et al. [16] studied the prevalence of dental traumatic injuries in children with a variety of SHCN and compared them to age- and gender-matched children who were typically developed. Overall, the prevalence of dental injuries in the children with SHCN was 8.7% while in the control subjects, it was 4.1%. The subjects were further identified by type of disability. Children with multiple disabilities were the most likely to experience dental traumatic injuries (14%), followed by children with intellectual disability (13.1%) and children with CP (12.2%) [45].

Holan et al. [46] evaluated a group of adolescents and young adults diagnosed with cerebral palsy who had cognitive ability within the range of normal. Clinical examinations were done to identify any signs of dental traumatic injury in the past. Fifty-seven percent of the study subjects demonstrated signs of dental traumatic injury.

1.4.8.3 Intellectual Disability

Children with intellectual disability and learning difficulties have been shown to be at increased risk for dental traumatic injuries. One reason for this may be that these children have other medical or developmental disorders that are linked to the cognitive abilities. In the study by Al-Batayneh et al. [16], children with intellectual disabilities had the second highest prevalence of dental injuries following children with multiple disabilities. This increased risk may be due to a lack of coordination or slower responses to objects in the environment.

### 1.4.9	Iatrogenic Injuries

Iatrogenic injuries consist of unintentional harm caused by medical or dental professionals in the process of providing care for some other medical condition. Intubation during a medical procedure and intubation for the management of the airway in a premature infant are two examples of this.

1.4.9.1 Prolonged Intubation of Neonate

Infants born prematurely are frequently intubated for a prolonged period due to immature lung development. The orotracheal tube is positioned in such a manner that it rests on the palate and maxillary alveolar ridge. This results in a depression in the alveolar ridge and may lead to enamel developmental defects in the primary teeth and potential damage to the tooth germs of the permanent teeth [47].

Some hospitals work with pediatric dentistry colleagues to fabricate an acrylic palatal stabilizing device that prevents groove formation, provides a slot for both the nasogastric tube and the orotracheal tube and minimizes the risk for accidental extubation in these extremely fragile neonates (Fig. 1.3) [48].

1.4.9.2 Intubation During General Anesthesia

Reports of perianesthetic dental injuries are variable and range from an incidence of 0.04–12% [47]. Newland et al., in a study of cases over a 14-year period, found an incidence of 1 dental injury per 2073 anesthesias [49]. The most common injuries were to the maxillary incisors and included fracture of the enamel, luxated, or avulsed teeth. Patients at the greatest risk for dental injury were those who were difficult to intubate and with poor dentition. In children, the dentition may be at risk because the primary teeth are decayed or close to exfoliation. The permanent

Fig. 1.3 The palatal stabilizing device is fabricated from an impression of the premature infant's maxilla while in the neonatal intensive care unit. It is made out of acrylic and covers the palate with grooves on the outer surface for the nasogastric tube and the oropharyngeal tube

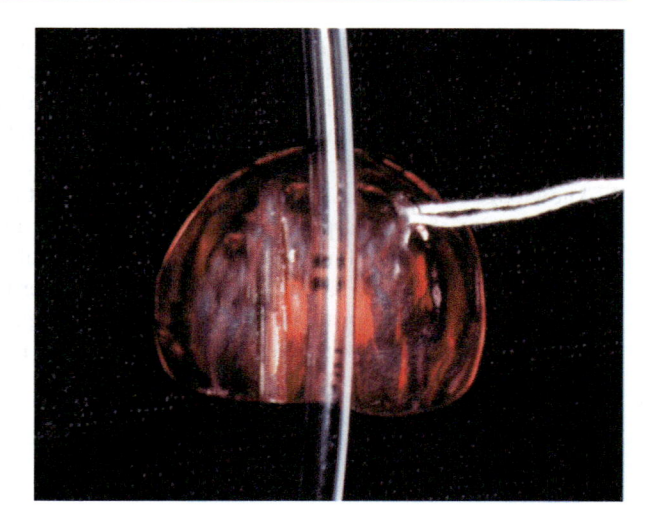

incisors may be at increased risk if they are newly erupted with incomplete root formation. Children who are obese or who have medical conditions that make intubation more challenging are also at greater risk for dental injury during intubation.

1.5   Treatment and Timing

The prognosis of traumatized teeth is intimately connected to the timeliness of treatment and the type of treatment provided. Evidence regarding the effective management of different types of TDIs has been used to develop guidelines for clinicians. These guidelines will be described in the next section. In addition to the guidelines, the timing of treatment is crucial. Many traumatic injuries occur in the evening after business hours or on the weekend when the patient's dental home is not open. Dental professionals are ethically responsible for the well-being of their patients and should have a protocol for managing after-hours emergencies. In the United States, it is rare for a local hospital to have the personnel or equipment to manage a dental emergency. University affiliated hospitals may have dental residency programs that provide after-hours care, but when these don't exist, dentists in private practice are responsible for providing this care. There is clear evidence that delay in providing care for TDIs results in a poor prognosis for the injured teeth. In a study comparing injuries to permanent teeth that occurred after-hours to those during office hours, Vukovic et al. reported that 90% of after-hours injuries had a median delay in treatment of 48 h [50]. Injuries that occurred during office hours had a median delay in treatment of 2.3 h. Significantly, more of the after-hours injuries resulted in complications including pulpitis, pulp necrosis, internal resorption, or extraction due to pulpal or periodontal complication.

A few studies have reported that some dentists choose to neglect providing treatment of TDIs in young children. When untreated traumatic injuries are observed, it is not always evident whether the parent chose not to bring the child to the dentist or that the dentist chose not to provide treatment. There is speculation that this lack of treatment is due to the perception by caregivers and health care providers that TDIs, particularly to primary teeth, do not require intervention. Since dentists receive limited training about the management of TDIs, it is possible that their lack of knowledge makes them hesitant to attempt treatment [51].

Studies also show a surprising lack of treatment for injuries to permanent anterior teeth. Marcenes et al. reported on a study of school children where more than half of the children who had experienced trauma to permanent maxillary incisors, had not been evaluated or treated by a dentist [52]. Again, it is unclear if this was due to caregivers not seeking care or not being able to find a dentist to provide the care.

1.6 Guidelines

The International Association for Dental Traumatology (IADT) [www.iadt-dental-trauma.org] has developed guidelines for the management of primary and permanent tooth trauma. They were developed by a working group of experienced researchers and clinicians and based on the best evidence available and on expert judgment if data was not available. The guidelines are updated on a regular basis as more data becomes available. The goal of the guidelines is to maximize the potential for positive outcomes. These guidelines have been endorsed by the American Academy of Pediatric Dentistry and the American Association of Endodontists and are available through the websites for these organizations or in the Journal Dental Traumatology [53–55].

The IADT also provides access for members to a number of other valuable resources. The Trauma Guide provides detailed information about examination of patients with TDIs, a Trauma Pathfinder to diagnose traumatic injuries and treatment guidelines for each type of injury separated by primary and permanent teeth. The IADT has recently developed an App for the iPhone and iPad that is free and available for professionals and patients. It includes the guidelines, helps identify the type of injury, and what should be done immediately to address the injury. It also provides a list of IADT member dentists.

References

1. Glendor U. Epidemiology of traumatic dental injuries–a 12 year review of the literature. Dent Traumatol. 2008;24:603–11.
2. Petti S, Glendor U, Andersson L. World traumatic dental injury prevalence and incidence, a meta-analysis-one billion living people have had traumatic dental injuries. Dent Traumatol. 2018;34:71–86.
3. Azami-Aghdash S, Azar EF, Azar PF, Rezapour A, Moradi-Joo M, Moosavi A, Oskouei GS. Prevalence, etiology, and types of dental trauma in children and adolescents: systematic review and meta-analysis. Med J Islam Repub Iran. 2015;29:234.

4. American Dental Association Commission on Dental Accreditation. Accreditation Standards for Advanced Dental Education Programs in Pediatric Dentistry. 2018. Chicago: American Dental Association. Adopted 8/3/2018. Implemented 1/1/2019 https://www.ada.org/~/media/CODA/Files/ped.pdf. Accessed 5/10/2019.

5. American Dental Association Commission on Dental Accreditation. Accreditation Standards for Advanced Dental Education Programs in Endodontics. 2018. Chicago: American Dental Association. Adopted 8/3/2018. Implemented 1/1/2019. https://www.ada.org/~/media/CODA/Files/endo.pdf. Accessed 5/10/2019.

6. Ravikuman D, Jeevanandan G, Subramanian EMG. Evaluation of knowledge among general dentists in treatment of traumatic injuries in primary teeth: a cross-sectional questionnaire study. Eur J Dent. 2017;11:232–7.

7. Hartmann RC, Rossetti BR, Siqueira Pinheiro L, Poli de Fiqueiredo JA, Rossi-Fedele G, S Gomes M, Gutierrez de Borba M. Dentists' knowledge of dental trauma based on the International Association of Dental Traumatology guidelines: a survey in South Brazil. Dent Traumatol. 2018; https://doi.org/10.1111/edt.12450. ahead of print.

8. Alyasi M, Al Halabi M, Hussein I, Khamis AH, Kowash M. Dentists' knowledge of the guidelines of traumatic dental injuries in the United Arab Emirates. Eur J Paediatr Dent. 2018;19:271–6.

9. Odersjo ML, Robertson A, Koch G. Incidence of dental traumatic injuries in children 0-4 years of age: a prospective study based on parental reporting. Eur Arch Paediatr Dent. 2018;19:107–11.

10. Flores MT, Holan G, Andreasen JO, Lauridsen E. Injuries to the primary dentition. In: Andreasen JO, Andreasen FM, Andersson L, editors. Textbook and color atlas of traumatic injuries to the teeth. 5th ed. Hoboken: Wiley-Blackwell; 2019. p. 556–88.

11. Fisher-Owens SA, Lukefahr JL, Tate AR, American Academy of Pediatrics, Section on Oral Health, Committee on Child Abuse and Neglect, American Academy of Pediatric Dentistry, Council on Clinical Affairs, Council on Scientific Affairs, Ad Hoc Work Group on Child Abuse and Neglect. Oral and dental aspects of child abuse and neglect. Pediatr Dent. 2017;39:278–83.

12. Sgan-Cohen HD, Megnagi G, Jacobi Y. Dental trauma and its association with anatomic, behavioral, and social variables among fifth and sixth grade schoolchildren in Jerusalem. Community Dent Oral Epidemiol. 2005;33:174–80.

13. Petti S. Over two hundred million injuries to anterior teeth attributable to large overjet: a meta-analysis. Dent Traumatol. 2015;31:1–8.

14. Herguner A, Erdur AE, Basciftci FA, Herguner S. Attention-deficit/hyperactivity disorder symptoms in children with traumatic dental injuries. Dent Traumatol. 2015;31:140–3.

15. Sabuncuoglu O, Irmak MY. 2017. The attention-deficit/hyperactivity disorder model for traumatic dental injuries: a critical review and update of the last 10 years. Dent Traumatol. 2017;33:71–6.

16. Al-Batayneh OB, Al O, Al-Saydali MO, Waldman HB. Traumatic dental injuries in children with special health care needs. Dent Traumatol. 2017;33:269–75.

17. Collins CL, McKenzie LB, Ferketich RA, Huiyun X, Comstock RD. Dental injuries sustained by high school athletes in the United States, from 2008/2009 through 2013/2014 academic years. Dent Traumatol. 2016;32:121–7.

18. Bakland LK. Traumatic dental injuries. In: Ingle JI, Bakland LK, editors. Endodontics. 5th ed. Baltimore: Williams & Wilkins; 2002. p. 795–844.

19. Cavalleri Z, Zerman N. Traumatic crown fractures in permanent incisors with immature roots: a follow-up study. Endod Dent Traumatol. 1995;11:294–6.

20. Borzabadi-Farahani A, Borzabadi-Farahani A, Eslamipour F. An investigation into the association between facial profile and maxillary incisor trauma, a clinical non-radiographic study. Dent Traumatol. 2010;26:403–8.

21. Bicycle Helmet Safety Institute. https://www.helmets.org/mandator.htm#international. Accessed 5/10/2019.

22. Chapman HR, Curran AL. Bicycle helmets—does the dental profession have a role in promoting their use? Br Dent J. 2004;196:555–60.

23. Thompson DC, Nunn ME, Thompson RS, Rivara F. Effectiveness of bicycle safety helmets in preventing serious facial injury. JAMA. 1996;276:1974–5.
24. Traffic Safety Facts 1997. National Highway Traffic Safety Administration, US Dept of Transportation; 1998. Publication DOT HS 808770.
25. National Center for Statistics and Analysis (NCSA) motor vehicle traffic crash data resource Page. https://crashstats.nhtsa.dot.gov/#/. Accessed 5/10/19.
26. Mouzakes J, Koltai PJ, Kuhar S, Bernstein DS, Wing P, Salsberg E. The impact of airbags and seat belts on the incidence and severity of maxillofacial injuries in automobile accidents in New York State. Arch Otolaryngol Head Neck Surg. 2001;127:1189–93.
27. Durbin DR, Chen I, Smith R, Elliott MR, Winston FK. Effects of seating position and appropriate restraint use on the risk of injury to children in motor vehicle crashes. Pediatrics. 2005;115:e305–9.
28. Natu SS, Pradhan H, Gupta H, Alam S, Gupta S, Pradhan R, Mohammad S, Kohli M, Sinha VP Shankar R, Agarwal A. An epidemiological study on pattern and incidence of mandibular fractures. Plast Surg Int. 2012;2012:834364.
29. World Health Organization fact sheet on child maltreatment. https://www.who.int/news-room/fact-sheets/detail/child-maltreatment. Accessed 12/28/18.
30. Centers for Disease Control and Prevention. Violence against children surveys: towards a violence-free generation. https://www.cdc.gov/violenceprevention/childabuseandneglect/vacs/index.html. Accessed 5/10/2019.
31. Child Welfare Information Gateway. Child abuse and neglect fatalities 2016: statistics and interventions. 2018. Children's Bureau/ACYF/ACF/HHS. https://www.childwelfare.gov/pub-PDFs/fatality.pdf. Accessed 12/28/18.
32. Christian CW, Committee on Child Abuse and Neglect, American Academy of Pediatrics. The evaluation of suspected child physical abuse. Pediatrics. 2015;135:e1337–54.
33. Ferreira MC, Batista AM, Ferreira FO, Ramos-Joege ML, Marques LS. Pattern of oral-maxillofacial trauma stemming from interpersonal physical violence and determinant factors. Dent Traumatol. 2014;30:15–21.
34. Gassner R, Bosch R, Tuli T, Emshoff R. Prevalence of dental trauma in 6000 patients with facial injuries: implications for prevention. Oral Surg Oral Med Oral Pathol Oral Radiol Endod. 1999;87:27–33.
35. Levin L, Lin S, Goldman S, Peleg K. Relationship between socio-economic position and general, maxillofacial and dental trauma: A National Trauma Registry Study. Dent Traumatol. 2010;26:342–5.
36. American College of Surgeons National Trauma Data Bank Pediatric Report 2016. https://www.facs.org/quality-programs/trauma/tqp/center-programs/ntdb/docpub. Accessed 12/7/18.
37. Dimitroulis G, Eyre J. A 7-year review of maxillofacial trauma in a central London hospital. Br Dent J. 1991;170:300–2.
38. ADHD Institute. https://adhd-institute.com/. Accessed 12/28/18.
39. Sabuncuoglu O, Taser H, Berkem M. Relationship between traumatic dental injuries and attention-deficit/hyperactivity disorder in children and adolescents: proposal of an explanatory model. Dent Traumatol. 2005;21:249–53.
40. Ziegler AM. Analysis of a comprehensive dental trauma database: an epidemiologic study of traumatic dental injuries to the permanent dentition. Dissertation, The Ohio State University; 2014.
41. Mayers LB, Chiffriller SH. Body art (body piercing and tattooing) among undergraduate university students: "then and now". J Adolesc Health. 2008;42:201–3.
42. Campbell A, Moore A, Williams E, Stephens J, Tatakis DN. Tongue piercing: impact of time and barbell stem length on lingual gingival recession and tooth chipping. J Periodontol. 2002;73:289–97.
43. Bessermann K. Frequency of maxillo-facial injuries in a hospital population of patients with epilepsy. Bull Nord Soc Dent Handicap. 1978;5:12–26.
44. Lagunju IA, Oyinlade AO, Babatunde OD. Seizure-related injuries in children and adolescents with epilepsy. Epilepsy Behav. 2016;54:131–4.

45. Cardoso AM, Silva CR, Gomes LN, Gomes MDAN, Padilha WW, Cavalcanti AL. Dental trauma in Brazilian children and adolescents with cerebral palsy. Dent Traumatol. 2015;31:471–6.
46. Holan G, Peretz B, Efrat J, Shapira Y. Traumatic injuries to the teeth in young individuals with cerebral palsy. Dent Traumatol. 2005;21:65–9.
47. Andersson L, Petti S, Day P, Kenny K, Glendor U, Andreasen JO. Classification, epidemiology and etiology. In: Andreasen JO, Andreasen FM, Andersson L, editors. Textbook and color atlas of traumatic injuries to the teeth. 5th ed. Hoboken: Wiley-Blackwell; 2019. p. 252–94.
48. Erenberg A, Nowak AJ. Appliance for stabilizing orogastric and orotracheal tubes in infants. Crit Care Med. 1984;12:669–71.
49. Newland MC, Ellis SJ, Peters KR, Simonson JA, Durham TM, Ullrich FA, Tinker JH. Dental injury associated with anesthesia: a report of 161,687 anesthetics given over 14 years. J Clin Anesth. 2007;19:339–45.
50. Vukovic A, Vukovic R, Markovic D, Soldatovic I, Mandinic Z, Beloica M, Stojan G. After-hours versus office-hours dental injuries in children: does timing influence outcome? Clin Pediatr. 2016;55:29–35.
51. Hamilton FA, Hill FJ, Holloway PJ. An investigation of dento-alveolar trauma and its treatment in an adolescent population. Part 2: dentists' knowledge of management methods and their perceptions of barriers to providing care. Br Dent J. 1997;182:129–33.
52. Marcenes W, Alessi ON, Traebert J. Causes and prevalence of traumatic injuries to the permanent incisors of school children aged 12 years in Jaragua do Sul, Brazil. Int Dent J. 2000;50:87–92.
53. DiAngelis AJ, Andreasen JO, Ebeleseder KA, Kenny DJ, Trope M, Sigurdsson A, Andersson L, Bourguignon C, Flores MT, Hicks ML, Lenzi AR, Malmgren B, Moule AJ, Pohl Y, Tsukiboshi M. Guidelines for the management of traumatic dental injuries: 1. Fractures and luxations of permanent teeth. Dent Traumatol. 2012;28:2–12.
54. Andersson L, Andreasen JO, Day P, Heithersay G, Trope M, DiAngelis AJ, Kenny DJ, Sigurdsson A, Bourguignon C, Flores MT, Hicks ML, Lenzi AR, Malmgren B, Moule AJ, Tsukiboshi M. Guidelines for the management of traumatic dental injuries: 2. Avulsion of permanent teeth. Dent Traumatol. 2012;28:88–96.
55. Malmgren B, Adreasen JO, Flores MT, Robertson A, DiAngelis AJ, Andersson L, Cavalleri G, Cohenca N, Day P, Hicks ML, Malmgren O, Moule AJ, Onetto J, Tsukiboshi M, International Association of Dental Traumatology. International Association of Dental Traumatology guidelines for the management of traumatic dental injuries: 3. Injuries in the primary dentition. Dent Traumatol. 2012;28:174–82.

Unique Challenges in the Pediatric Population

2

Pediatric patients present a unique challenge to oral health care providers for a variety of reasons. First, depending on their age, maturity, temperament, and developmental status, their behavior may make treatment in the traditional dental setting difficult. Second, young children may not be able to accurately describe their symptoms or details of how an injury occurred. Third, children and adolescents require a parent or caregiver to provide consent for treatment, adding additional people who need to be involved in the communication. Some children may be in foster care and it may be unclear if the foster parent can provide consent for treatment. Fourth, caregivers may have strong opinions about what treatment should be provided and this may go against current accepted guidelines. Fifth, children and their dentitions are in a constant state of growth and development and these factors need to be considered in any treatment plan. Finally, it is incumbent on the health care provider to determine if the injury matches the description provided or if there is a potential concern for child abuse or maltreatment.

2.1 Behavior Guidance

Techniques to guide a patient through an invasive dental procedure are based on the child's age and developmental maturity. Knowledge and effective use of these techniques is a vital component of pediatric dentistry training programs and a skill that often sets the pediatric dentist apart from general dentists. Because this is such an important component of the practice of pediatric dentistry, the American Academy of Pediatric Dentistry (AAPD) sponsored the first symposium on behavior management in 1988. The outcome of that symposium was the development of the first guidelines on this topic. Subsequently, the AAPD sponsored additional symposia focused on behavior guidance in 2003 and 2013 which informed updates to the behavior guidance document [1]. This document is available through the AAPD website and published annually in the AAPD Reference Manual.

© Springer Nature Switzerland AG 2020
R. L. Slayton, E. A. Palmer, *Traumatic Dental Injuries in Children*,
https://doi.org/10.1007/978-3-030-25793-4_2

At very young ages (generally under 3 years), children may be described as "pre-cooperative". This implies that it is unreasonable to expect the toddler to sit in a dental chair and cooperate for a stranger to examine or treat a dental condition or injury. There are certainly exceptions where young children have surprisingly good coping skills or where older children have limited ability to cope.

Pediatric dentists spend a significant portion of their specialty training learning how to manage a child's behavior so that preventive and restorative care can be accomplished in the traditional dental setting. This includes non-pharmacologic techniques such as Tell-Show-Do, distraction, positive reinforcement, and voice control among others. When those techniques are not successful, more advanced methods such as protective stabilization, procedural sedation, and general anesthesia are considered. All of these methods require communication with the caregiver and either verbal or written informed consent.

In many parts of the United States and the world, there is limited access to a pediatric dentist. General dentists are often put in the position of needing to provide care for challenging patients in difficult situations. Stabilizing the patient's injury so that they can be transported to the office of a pediatric dentist to provide definitive care, may be in the child's best interest, depending on the severity of the injury and the experience of the dentist with young children.

Traumatic dental injuries by definition, occur unexpectedly and for young children, may be the reason for their first dental visit. This limits the dentist's ability to establish rapport and gain trust from the child and caregivers. There is an urgency to provide treatment and emotions are high. From the dentist's perspective, the injury often occurs after-hours and since traumatic injuries may be relatively uncommon in his or her practice, it is difficult to be prepared for whatever may have happened. Having easily accessible reference materials and a "trauma kit" to manage the majority of traumatic dental injuries will allow the dentist to provide care in a confident, effective manner.

Many of the recommendations for ways to make the dental environment comfortable for children and families rely on being able to plan ahead for the child's visit. This includes things like scheduling the appointment for earlier in the day, giving the child a chance to visit the office prior to having any invasive procedures, letting the family meet the dental team and having the opportunity to communicate with the caregiver about mutual expectations. When the child's first visit is for a traumatic injury, most of these protocols are put on hold and the focus is on addressing the injury. Even for patients of record, the traumatic injury may be the first time the child is facing the need for an invasive procedure. The dentist must have a full set of behavior guidance tools to use and be skilled at determining what will be most effective for the patient in the current situation. The considerations for behavior guidance at the time of a traumatic injury are discussed below in order from least to most complex.

2.2 Behavior Guidance Considerations

Basic behavior guidance techniques are considered to be the starting point for managing the behavior of a child during a dental visit. They primarily involve communicating with the child in a way that is appropriate for their level of development.

For example, toddlers should be given one request at a time while an older child may be able to understand a series of requests. Establishing trust and rapport is important when treating a young child and even during an emergency situation, this can be accomplished by the dentist appearing calm and confident and using words that don't sound threatening. The AAPD has developed a guideline on behavior guidance that provides details about each of the techniques described below [1]. The most commonly used techniques are described. Other less commonly used techniques are described in the AAPD guidelines [1].

2.2.1 Tell-Show-Do

Tell-Show-Do is a commonly used technique that is nonthreatening and simple for a dentist to learn. The dentist describes what is going to happen, shows a picture of it or demonstrates it on a model and then performs the procedure on the child. This technique relies on the use of "child friendly" words instead of the typical dental terminology. The slow speed handpiece is commonly referred to as "Mr. Bumpy" and the high-speed handpiece as "Mr. Whistle." Local anesthetic may be referred to as "sleepy water." The dentist can show the child how the prophy cup feels on their fingernail or let them hear the sound of the high-speed handpiece. This technique is well accepted by children and caregivers and is relatively easy for a dentist to learn and implement [2].

2.2.2 Positive Reinforcement

Positive reinforcement is another non-pharmacologic technique that can be very effective for some children. This technique relies on the dentist recognizing when the child is being cooperative and providing positive comments about that behavior. Even when the child is not behaving perfectly, there is usually some part of their behavior that is cooperative and worthy of comment. If the child is lying still, opening their mouth for the exam or following instructions, those are all behaviors that should be noticed and commented on. Positive comments are particularly effective when said in front of caregivers.

Other forms of positive reinforcement include providing the child with a sticker or a small toy at the end of the appointment. Sometimes the anticipation of this prize helps the child cooperate during the procedure [2].

2.2.3 Distraction

Some children respond very well to distraction techniques. When done effectively, it can keep the child's mind off of the procedure and help them to cope. Distraction techniques may involve telling the child a story or singing a song while giving an injection or initiating a painful procedure. Having the child focus on spelling out their name with their foot or thinking of what they want to do when they get home can also serve as a distraction. In some of the more recently built dental operatories and in the emergency rooms of Children's Hospitals, the use of cartoons on overhead televisions has been very useful to distract and calm children before and during invasive procedures.

2.2.4 Voice Control

Voice control is an effective way to achieve compliance from a child if it is used appropriately. This technique involves modifying the tone or volume of the voice to get the child's attention and to make it clear what the expectations are. It is important that the facial expression mirrors the message being delivered [3]. The voice should be firm and positive, not loud and emotional. When the child responds to the request, positive reinforcement should be provided. Although this is an effective technique, it is viewed by some caregivers as aversive. Parenting styles vary considerably in the U.S. and other countries. If the caregiver views voice control as "yelling" at their child, they may object to its use. When feasible, describing this technique in advance and getting "buy in" from the caregiver may be effective in eliminating or minimizing misunderstandings.

2.2.5 Escape

Escape is a technique that can be effective for some children and may be useful in situations where a traumatic injury has occurred. This is a technique that allows the child to "take a break" from the procedure. Two types of escape have been described in the literature [2]. The first is "contingent escape." This is given to the patient when they are cooperative for a procedure. For example, the child is told they can take a break if they keep their mouth open until the count of 10. Studies of this type of management have shown it to be nonaversive and effective for preschool-aged children [4]. Noncontingent escape is also effective and involves giving the child a break without any expectations of behavior change. This could be as simple as the dentist leaving the room to check on another patient but telling the child to take a break for a few minutes until he or she returns.

When treating a traumatic dental injury, time is often crucial, so incorporating breaks into the treatment protocol may not be practical.

2.2.6 Parent Presence

Parent (or caregiver) presence (or absence) is considered a form of behavior guidance. It is somewhat controversial, and its use varies from one dentist to the next. Many pediatric dentists were trained to believe that a child will be more cooperative for care if the caregiver is not in the operatory. This gives the dentist the opportunity to communicate directly with the child and to establish trust and rapport without having to "compete" with the caregiver for the child's attention. Those who favor having the caregiver in the operatory, value the ability to communicate with the caregiver about findings of the exam throughout the visit and are able to set boundaries for the caregiver during the visit. Some also believe that having the caregiver present may improve the child's behavior if the child is told that the caregiver can stay as long as the child is cooperative. It is important that caregivers understand in advance that they may be asked to leave the operatory. This can be a source of conflict and may make the situation worse if it is not agreed to in advance. In a study of parental presence in uncooperative child dental patients, Boka et al. found no difference between children who had a parent present in the operatory and children without a parent present [5]. At the time of treating a traumatic injury, having a parent or caregiver present is important to help calm the child, to obtain information about the traumatic event and to get informed consent for the treatment proposed.

2.2.7 Deferred Treatment

Deferred treatment is considered to be a form of behavior guidance when the child's behavior makes treatment unsafe and the treatment needs are not urgent [1]. This could be used in some types of traumatic injuries, particularly if there is a safe way to stabilize the injury. Providing definitive treatment in an after-hours setting is rarely ideal. In the office setting after-hours, the dentist may be alone and may not have access to all of the necessary supplies and equipment that would be available during business hours. Some hospital emergency rooms are equipped to handle dental emergencies, but many are only able to provide palliative care at the time of the injury. When a dental injury can be managed with minimal treatment to stabilize the tooth until regular office hours, this allows the child to get a good night's sleep and recover from the traumatic experience. This is not an option for more severe traumatic injuries but should be considered an option for the less severe cases.

2.2.8 Nitrous Oxide

Nitrous oxide inhalation is included in basic behavior guidance techniques but is also considered mild sedation [6]. It is very effective in reducing anxiety in children and is useful for operative procedures as well as treatment of traumatic injuries. Most pediatric dentistry practices in the U.S. have access to nitrous oxide in some or all of their operatories. Some hospitals, particularly those with pediatric dentistry or oral and maxillofacial surgery residencies, have at least one room in the emergency department that is equipped with nitrous oxide. In order for nitrous oxide to be effective, the child must be able to tolerate the nasal hood and breathe through their nose. Excessive crying interferes with the effectiveness of this agent because instead of reaching the lungs, the gas is expelled through the mouth. When used appropriately, it is effective at managing anxiety and uncooperative behavior and is generally well accepted by children and caregivers.

When using any type of sedation, it is important to have the appropriate training and to follow established guidelines for administration, monitoring and follow-up. The AAPD in collaboration with the American Academy of Pediatrics established guidelines for the monitoring and management of pediatric patients before, during, and after sedation [7]. Established in 2006, the guideline was recently updated to clarify monitoring methods and techniques to improve safety. The AAPD also has a guideline on the use of nitrous oxide that provides additional information about when and how this inhalation agent should be used [6].

Dentists should be familiar with the training requirements and regulations governing the use of nitrous oxide in their state or country. In some U.S. states, a separate sedation permit is required in addition to the dental license.

Important contraindications for the use of nitrous oxide include: current upper respiratory infection [8], recent middle ear infection or surgery [8], severe methylenetetrahydrofolate reductase (MTHFR) deficiency, [9] and Cobalamin (vitamin B-12) deficiency [10].

Nitrous oxide systems are designed with a fail-safe function so that there is never less than 30% oxygen supplied with the nitrous oxide. When used with children, a nitrous concentration of 35–50% is both safe and effective. The two methods of induction are either by slow titration, where the concentration of nitrous oxide is increased over a 4–5 min time period or rapid, where the concentration is set to the desired level between 35 and 50% immediately.

Nitrous oxide inhalation may be very useful for the management of traumatic dental injuries because it is effective in managing painful procedures and anxiety. However, because the nasal hood rests on the upper lip and because many dental injuries involve the maxillary teeth, the use of nitrous oxide might not be practical.

A child with good coping skills and one who trusts that the dentist is there to help them is likely to be cooperative for treatment in the traditional dental setting using non-pharmacologic techniques or with the addition of nitrous oxide.

2.3   Advanced Behavior Guidance Techniques

Advanced behavior guidance techniques include protective stabilization and pharmacologic management with mild or moderate sedation and general anesthesia. These techniques require specific training and licensure and should only be performed according to established guidelines. The safety of the child should always be the primary consideration.

2.3.1   Protective Stabilization

This technique is described as: "the physical limitation of a patient's movement by a person or restrictive equipment, materials or devices for a finite period of time in order to safely provide examination, diagnosis, and/or treatment" [11]. When a device is used, such as a safety wrap (Fig. 2.1), it is considered passive

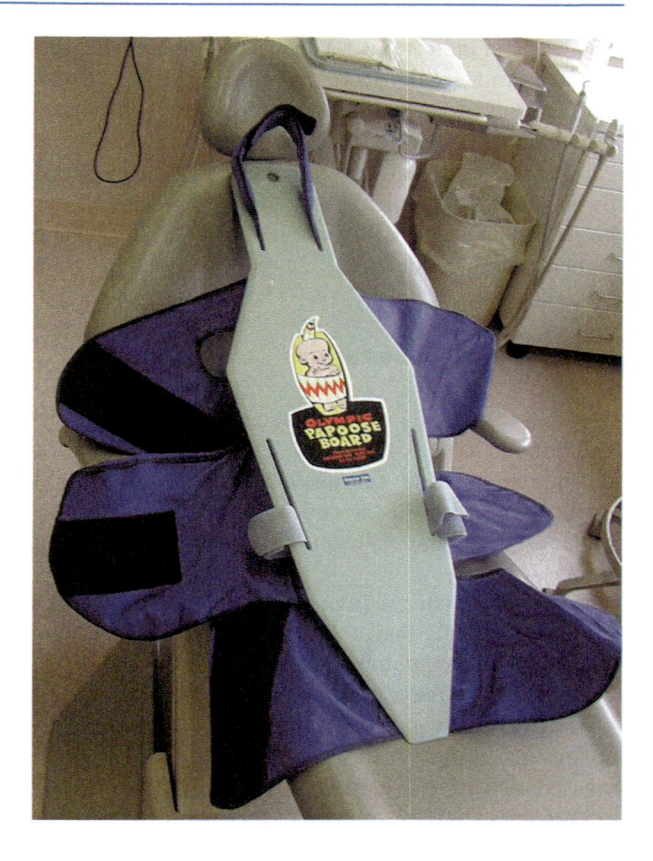

Fig. 2.1 In some situations, a stability wrap may be used to protect and stabilize the child so that an urgent procedure can be completed. The blue material wraps around the child's shoulders, torso and legs and is secured with Velcro. Consent must be obtained from the caregiver and documented in the dental record

immobilization. When the restraint is performed by a person holding the hands or legs, it is considered active immobilization.

Proper training for dentists and their staff is crucial in order to avoid injury to the patient and providers. In most dental schools, students have limited exposure to this technique. It is an essential part of pediatric dentistry specialty training.

Use of protective stabilization requires informed consent from a parent or legal guardian. Informed consent means that the procedure is explained in detail, including the risks, benefits, and alternatives so that the caregiver can make an informed decision about how to proceed. It is preferable for this discussion and the consent to be obtained on a day prior to the procedure. At the time of a traumatic dental injury, this may not be possible, since treatment may be required urgently. The information provided and signed consent should be documented in the patient record prior to beginning treatment [11]. Laws concerning informed consent vary by state. Dentists should be aware of the laws in their state and document accordingly.

In addition to the documentation related to the consent process, the dentist and/or their staff should document the reason for the use of protective stabilization, type of device used, length of time used, behavior during the procedure, any unexpected outcomes or injuries, and suggestions for future appointments [11].

The main indications for the use of protective stabilization in cases of traumatic dental injuries are the need for urgent, limited treatment for a child that is not able to cooperate due to their age, anxiety, or emotional status. In this situation, it facilitates the safe treatment of the child so that the necessary treatment can be completed.

The use of protective stabilization is not recommended for cooperative patients or patients with medical or psychological conditions that could be harmed by the protective device. It is also not indicated for non-emergent treatment or for the convenience of the dentist [11].

2.3.2 Minimal Sedation

Minimal sedation is a drug-induced state in which the patient can still understand and respond to verbal requests. It does not result in impairment of cardiovascular or respiratory function. In most cases, minimal sedation is accomplished using oral medications with the exception of nitrous oxide inhalation anesthesia (discussed previously) and midazolam (versed) which can be administered orally, intranasally, or intravenously.

Many U.S. states require additional training and licensure to administer sedative agents to patients under 12 years of age. It is incumbent on each provider to be familiar with the guidelines in their state or country.

The primary purpose of minimal sedation is to reduce anxiety related to a dental procedure. This can be very useful for the management of traumatic dental injuries so long as appropriate guidelines are followed. In particular, the child must meet the pre-sedation criteria described in the AAPD Guidelines [7]. Children should be American Society of Anesthesiologists (ASA) classification I or II, have had nothing to eat for 6 h, clear liquids up to 2 h prior to procedure, no evidence of upper respiratory infection, and determined to have adequate airway.

It is essential that the appropriate qualified staff are available to monitor the patient and that the facilities include the necessary equipment to manage any potential emergencies during or after the procedure. There is always the possibility that a patient will become more deeply sedated than intended. The dental team should be prepared to manage the deeper level of sedation until the patient returns to the intended level.

Detailed documentation of the sedation on a separate form is crucial. The AAPD Reference Manual includes a sample form that can be adapted for use by member dentists [AAPD Sedation Record] [https://www.aapd.org/research/oral-health-policies%2D%2Drecommendations/sedation-record/] This record serves as a reminder for doses of reversal drugs, provides a chart of the vital signs during the procedure and serves as documentation regarding the level of success the medication (s) provided.

Sedating a child in an office setting after-hours should be considered carefully to ensure that the safety of the child and the dental staff members is maintained. If sedation cannot be safely performed in the office setting, the patient should be transferred to the local emergency department or provided with palliative care until the next day during normal office hours.

2.3.3 Moderate Sedation

Moderate sedation is a drug-induced condition in which patients are able to respond to requests with light tactile stimulation. Loss of consciousness is unlikely unless they have reached a state of deep sedation unintentionally. The airway and cardiovascular functions are not compromised during moderate sedation. When moderate sedation is used, the patient should be continuously monitored with a pulse oximeter. The respiratory rate and blood pressure should be monitored and recorded intermittently.

Medications used for moderate sedation are generally given orally or intranasally and may be used in combination. Vital signs, doses given, and other relevant information should be recorded on a sedation record, such as that provided by the AAPD. The dental team should be prepared to manage the patient at the deep sedation level, which means that the appropriate emergency medications and equipment should be available in the event that the patient becomes more deeply sedated than intended [7].

If a child requires moderate sedation after-hours to manage a traumatic dental injury, it is recommended that the patient be transferred to the local hospital emergency department unless the treatment can be delayed until normal office hours.

2.3.4 General Anesthesia

General anesthesia produces a state of unconsciousness and a loss of protective reflexes. Patients under general anesthesia cannot maintain their airway and are generally intubated or assisted in some way. Most pediatric dentists do not have the necessary training to administer general anesthesia and rely on anesthesiologists practicing in a hospital or in an office-based practice. For patients with severe dental or maxillofacial trauma and for very young children or children with special health care needs (SHCN), treatment under general anesthesia may be warranted. This creates a challenging situation because the operating rooms in most hospitals are tightly scheduled and may not be able to accommodate a dental injury on short notice. Pediatric dentists with hospital privileges can coordinate this care when needed but, in some cases, the child must be transported to a tertiary care facility that is affiliated with a university- or hospital-based residency program.

2.4 Consent

As mentioned previously, consent for treatment of children and adolescents must be provided by the legal guardian. It is important to determine the status of the adult who is accompanying the child following a traumatic injury. Situations may be encountered where divorced parents share custody and both need to agree on treatment; foster parents who may not have detailed information about the child's medical history; a child's nanny or an older sibling who may have permission to bring the child to an appointment but not to consent for invasive treatment. It is essential to understand the relationship of the person accompanying the child patient and to document this in the patient record. Consent may need to be obtained over the phone and if possible, another person should be on the line as a witness to what was agreed to.

2.5   Communication

Clear, patient-centered communication regarding the findings and recommended treatment must be provided to the patient and caregiver so that an informed decision can be made about the treatment and follow-up care. There are usually multiple options to consider, so describing these in a way that families understand is crucial. Avoiding medical or dental terminology will help with this.

It has been estimated that by 2020, 40% of school-aged children will be from a minority group [12]. This has implications for cultural differences as well as language and communication issues. In the U.S., 63 million people speak a language other than English at home and more than 26 million have very limited ability to understand English [13]. Language barriers have been shown to impact access to health care, communication with health care providers, satisfaction with care, and patient safety [13, 14]. Qualified interpreters are essential for communicating information about diagnosis and treatment options and to obtain an accurate medical history for a child patient. However, it is often challenging to find an interpreter with the specific language skills needed for an after-hours emergency in a non-hospital setting. In the U.S., there are many interpreters that can be accessed by phone and some of the new programs for translation may help on short notice but are not ideal for managing a complex traumatic injury. Computer programs such as Google Translate may be helpful for simple communication needs but are not practical for medical informed consent.

Additional communication challenges exist when a child has a complex medical condition or other SHCN. In 2007, Wise estimated that 16% of children in the United States had SHCN [15]. At that time, 13% of children with SHCN lived in homes where English was not the primary language [15]. More recently, the CDC reported that 1 in 5 children in the United States has a special health care need [16]. The increase in children with SHCN and families with limited English proficiency creates unique opportunities for medical and dental providers when caring for urgent traumatic injuries.

2.6   Parental Presence

The decision to have caregivers present during treatment of a child is something that each dentist has to decide for themselves. Modern day parents are more likely to want to be present than in the past and in emergency situations, a parent or caregiver is often a calming influence, especially for young children. There are a number of advantages to having caregivers present during treatment of a traumatic injury. Since young children are not good historians, the caregivers are relied upon to provide details of the injury, medical and dental history, immunization history and other relevant factors that will influence treatment decisions. Having the caregiver present gives them the opportunity to provide support and encouragement to their child and to observe the treatment being provided so that they are more confident in the ability of the dentist and their staff. Having the caregiver present may also make informed consent more efficient if treatment needs to be modified as additional findings are discovered [1].

In some situations, it is not practical or advisable for caregivers to be present. This may be the case if the caregiver is very anxious and displaying disruptive behavior or if the child needs to be treated under sedation or general anesthesia. Communication with the caregiver about how treatment will be managed is an important part of the informed consent discussion.

2.7 Growth and Development Considerations

Providing treatment to a patient whose dentition is in a constant state of change creates a unique challenge, especially when a traumatic dental injury is involved. When a child in the primary dentition has a traumatic dental injury, one of the first considerations (after medical concerns) is the risk of injury to the developing permanent teeth. In some situations, the primary tooth is sacrificed in order to minimize damage to the permanent tooth. When it is reasonable to retain a primary tooth that has been injured, the goal is to maintain it until normal exfoliation. This may be a few years rather than a lifetime for permanent teeth.

In the mixed dentition, if a permanent incisor is avulsed or luxated and requires splinting as part of the management, it is likely that adjacent primary teeth are close to exfoliation and not reasonable anchorage for a splint. This may require extending the splint to the permanent molars. Careful evaluation of the timing of exfoliation of existing teeth is an important consideration. In this cohort, it is also likely that the incisors are only partially developed. Teeth with open apices have the possibility of pulp regeneration after a traumatic dental injury and it is essential that the treatment provided facilitates this process when possible.

Adolescents with complete permanent dentition may still have teeth with an open apex that need to be managed in a way that facilitates pulp regeneration. In addition, children in this age group may be in some stage of orthodontic treatment. In this case, it is often necessary to remove bands and brackets so that appropriate treatment of the TDI can be accomplished. If the dentist treating the patient does not have the instruments or expertise to remove orthodontic appliances, the child's orthodontist should be contacted to do this emergently.

2.8 Child Abuse

Any injury that doesn't match the description given has the potential to be the result of child abuse. Careful evaluation of the injury and the history given should be performed. Although the most common age for non-accidental dental injuries is between 2 and 4 years, it can occur at any age [17].

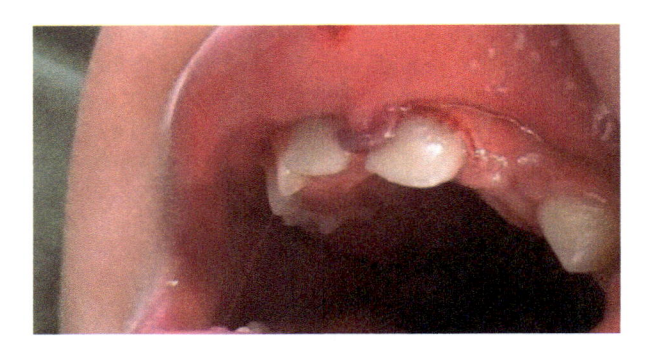

Fig. 2.2 It is not uncommon for a child to have a torn labial frenum as the result of a fall. Since this may also be an indication of child maltreatment, the details surrounding the traumatic incident should be thoroughly investigated. (Courtesy of the University of Iowa Pediatric Dentistry Department)

More than half of child abuse cases involve craniofacial, head, face, and neck injuries. This includes lacerations to the tongue, gingiva, and mucosa, fractured, luxated or avulsed teeth or fractured jaws [18].

One of the signs that most physicians and dentists were taught to consider as a possible indicator of child abuse is a torn labial frenum (Fig. 2.2). Although this finding should not be dismissed, and can be a sign of abuse, it is also important to note that studies on this topic have shown that a torn labial frenum in isolation is not pathognomonic for abuse. Teece and Crawford (2005) reviewed 104 papers and concluded that there was no evidence of the sensitivity and specificity for a torn frenum in a child being a sign of a non-accidental injury [19].

References

1. American Academy of Pediatric Dentistry. Behavior guidance for the pediatric dental patient. Pediatr Dent. 2018;40(special issue):254–67.
2. Townsend JA, Wells MH. Behavior guidance of the pediatric dental patient. In: Nowak AJ, Christensen JR, Mabry TR, Townsend JA, Wells MH, editors. Pediatric dentistry infancy through adolescence. Philadelphia: Elsevier; 2019. p. 352–70.
3. Pinkham JR, Patterson JR. Voice control: an old technique reexamined. ASDC J Dent Child. 1985;52:199–202.
4. Allen KD, Loiben T, Allen SJ, Stanley RT. Dentist-implemented contingent escape for management of disruptive child behavior. J Appl Behav Anal. 1992;25:629–36.
5. Boka V, Arapostathis K, Charitoudis G, Veerkamp J, van Loveren C, Kotsanos N. A study of parental presence/absence technique for child dental behaviour management. Eur Arch Paediatr Dent. 2017;18:405–9.
6. American Academy of Pediatric Dentistry. Use of nitrous oxide for pediatric dental patients. Pediatr Dent. 2018;40(special issue):281–6.
7. American Academy of Pediatric Dentistry. Monitoring and management of pediatric patients before, during and after sedation for diagnostic and therapeutic procedures: update 2016. Pediatr Dent. 2018;40(special issue):287–316.
8. Clark MS, Brunick AL. N$_2$O and its interaction with the body. In: Handbook of nitrous oxide and oxygen sedation, vol. 2015. 4th ed. St. Louis: Elsevier Mosby. p. 90–8.

9. Selzer RR, Rosenblatt DS, Laxova R, Hogan K. Adverse effect of nitrous oxide in a child with 5,10-methylenetetrahydrofolate reductase deficiency. N Engl J Med. 2003;349:45–50.
10. Sanders RDB, Weimann J, Maze M. Biologic effects of nitrous oxide: a mechanistic and toxicologic review. Anesthesiology. 2008;109:707–22.
11. American Academy of Pediatric Dentistry. Protective stabilization for pediatric dental patients. Pediatr Dent. 2018;40(special issue):268–73.
12. Harper DC, D'Allesandro DM. The child's voice: understanding the contexts of children and families today. Pediatr Dent. 2004;26:114–20.
13. Mosquera RA, Samuels C, Flores G. Family language barriers and special-needs children. Pediatrics. 2016;138:e20160321. https://doi.org/10.1542/peds.2016-0321.
14. Flores G, Abreu M, Barone CP, Bachur R, Lin H. Errors of medical interpretation and their potential clinical consequences: a comparison of professional versus ad hoc versus no interpreters. Ann Emerg Med. 2012;60:545–53.
15. Wise PH. The future pediatrician: the challenge of chronic illness. J Pediatr. 2007;151(Suppl 5):S6–S10.
16. Centers for Disease Control and Prevention. Children and youth with special healthcare needs in emergencies. https://www.cdc.gov/childrenindisasters/children-with-special-healthcare-needs.html. Accessed 1/7/19.
17. American Society for the Positive Care of Children. https://americanspcc.org/child-abuse-statistics/. Accessed 12/28/18.
18. Fisher-Owens SA, Lukefahr JL, Tate AR, American Academy of Pediatrics, Section on Oral Health, Committee on Child Abuse and Neglect, American Academy of Pediatric Dentistry, Council on Clinical affairs, Council on Scientific Affairs, Ad Hoc Work Group on Child Abuse and Neglect. Oral and dental aspects of child abuse and neglect. Pediatr Dent. 2017;39(4):278–83.
19. Teece S, Crawford I. Best evidence topic report. Torn frenulum and non-accidental injury in children. Emerg Med J. 2005;22:125.

Physical Examination and Diagnosis

3

When a child presents with a traumatic dental injury, it is paramount that thorough documentation is made of the event, treatment, and follow-up. It is best to follow a consistent format during acute trauma appointments in order to prevent overlooking key information and to establish a complete and correct diagnosis of all soft and hard tissue injuries [1–4]. One method is with the use of an assessment form that includes all of the information to be gathered. A sample assessment form entitled "Assessment of Acute Traumatic Injuries" published by the American Academy of Pediatric Dentistry can be found at http://www.aapd.org/media/Policies_Guidelines/R_AcuteTrauma.pdf [5]. The injury should also be documented with clinical photographs and radiographs as indicated. An additional challenge for the dentist will be managing a child's traumatic dental injury in combination with any complex medical history, special health care needs, and/or behavioral difficulties.

3.1 Initial Assessment

A child that presents to the dental office for emergency treatment of a dental injury may also have experienced more extensive oral, facial, and/or head trauma. It is not expected that the dentist would treat head injuries, but it is important that he/she recognizes the symptoms of possible neurologic involvement and refers the patient for appropriate care. Only after the provider has assessed the child's neurologic status, should the dental injury be addressed.

Often the initial contact with the family following a traumatic dental injury is over the phone. The front office staff or after-hours service should be provided with a script to help them assess the urgency of the injury and if the family should be directed to the emergency department or the dental office for care.

© Springer Nature Switzerland AG 2020
R. L. Slayton, E. A. Palmer, *Traumatic Dental Injuries in Children*,
https://doi.org/10.1007/978-3-030-25793-4_3

Triage script for front desk or after-hours call service
How old is your child?
Did the child lose consciousness?
If a tooth was knocked out, was it found?
When did the accident happen?
How did the accident happen?
Who witnessed the accident?
Where did the accident happen?

The physical assessment of the child should begin as soon as the child enters the dental office.

As the child and caregiver enter the dental office, the dental provider should greet the patient and make rapid observations about the following [6]:

1. Overall presentation:
   - Is the child fully ambulatory or requiring assistance to stand or walk?
   - Does the child have regular or abnormal respiratory rate or rhythm?
   - Are there any signs of lethargy, confusion, and/or drowsiness?
2. Altered cerebral function:
   - Does the child have an unusual verbal response?
   - Has the child been experiencing nausea or vomiting?
   - Is there asymmetry or decreased reaction of the pupils?
   - Is there evidence of bleeding or clear fluid from the nose or ears?
   - Is there abnormal position or movement of the eyes?
3. Obvious injuries to the face and head:
   - Does the child have facial bruising, abrasions, contusions, or lacerations that are evident?

These findings can be used to complete the Modified Glasgow Coma Scale [7]. If injuries to the face and/or head are noted in combination with signs or symptoms of a compromised overall presentation or altered mental status, the presence of neurological problems are possible. If at this point, the dental provider suspects neurological trauma, immediate dental treatment is contraindicated and the patient should be referred to the emergency room for comprehensive medical and neurological examination [6].

During the initial assessment, the dental provider will also be able to make some initial behavioral assessments about the child. If the child is being carried by the caregiver with their face hidden in the caregiver's shoulder, it is a good indication that the dental team will need to use some behavior management techniques (see Chap. 2 for details) in order to help the child to complete the assessment.

3.2   Patient/Family Interview

Following the initial assessment, the dental provider must gain an understanding of the injury itself. Using the AAPD trauma assessment form as a guide, the provider should interview the child and adult [5]. The child and adult should each recount what happened to cause the injury in their own words. Discrepancies between the stories may be suggestive of a non-accidental injury. Depending on the child's ability to communicate and articulate himself/herself, information about the injury may need to come from the adult accompanying the child. If the accompanying adult is unable to provide the necessary information, it is preferential to speak with someone more familiar with the child's injury via the telephone. The details of what happened, where and when the injury occurred, and treatment delivered since the injury should be recorded. These questions will provide information that will help direct the course of treatment. If the injury occurred outdoors, it is possible that the lesions were contaminated with unclean soil and the need for tetanus immunization could be important. Having an understanding of how the injury occurred may provide information regarding the other tissues likely affected in addition to the primary tissues impacted, e.g., a direct chin impact can result in condylar fractures as well as posterior tooth fractures. The time elapsed since the injury occurred is essential information in several injury types, e.g., avulsion. The patient should also be asked about any disturbances in his/her bite which could indicate an alveolar, jaw, or condylar fracture or a displaced tooth. It is important to ask about any systemic side effects such as loss of consciousness, headache, nausea and/or vomiting, altered orientation/mental status, dizziness, or blurred vision, and pain as a result of the injury. If there is any concern for a possible undiagnosed systemic condition, the patient should be evaluated in the emergency room immediately.

3.3   Medical History

A thorough medical history should be obtained. For a patient of record, that will be fairly straightforward with updates to the already known information including new medications, allergies, and tetanus immunization status. It is also important to ask about a history of previous trauma to the head, neck, or mouth. For new patients to the practice, a comprehensive medical history that includes all systemic diagnoses, recent hospitalizations, allergies and medications must also be gathered. A medical consultation may be indicated prior to treatment for any patient with significant cardiac conditions, immunocompromised status, or bleeding concerns. In such a case in which a medical consult is required prior to treatment and the medical provider is not available to speak via telephone, it would be prudent to triage and minimally stabilize the injury until the desired consult is obtained.

Information about the patient's dental history should also be gathered. The caregiver should be asked if the child has any behavioral or sensory challenges. If so, then a follow-up discussion should ensue in which the child's triggers are identified as well as the tools with which the child uses best to cope. This is also a good time to share the dentist's approach to behavior management. The dentist and caregiver can then develop a strategy in which to proceed. Consent for advanced behavior management, such as protective stabilization, can be given at this time.

3.4   Neurologic Evaluation

The child should initially undergo a neurological evaluation. First, the child's responsiveness should be assessed to insure that it is appropriate for their age and time of day at which the exam is occurring. Each cranial nerve should also be evaluated for proper function (Table 3.1) [5, 8]. If the child exhibits any symptoms (e.g., headache), physical signs (e.g., unsteadiness), impaired brain function (e.g., confusion), or abnormal behavior, a concussion should be suspected. All children with an aberrant neurological evaluation must be immediately examined by a medical team trained in neurological injuries.

Table 3.1 Cranial nerve examination for a child

Cranial nerve	Type of test	Instruct child to…	When to be concerned
I Olfactory	Smell test using peppermint, berry, orange, or chocolate smelling items	Close their eyes and identify what they are smelling	Child is unable to smell or name the smell
II Optic	Visual fields test to (1) evaluate pupil size (2) determine visual acuity using a chart with different colored letters	(1) Look at provider's nose (2) Identify colors or letters pointed to on the chart	(1) Unequal pupil size, symmetry (2) Unable to identify different colors or letters
III Oculomotor IV Trochlear VI Abducens	Extraocular movements to test (1) Pupil size and reactivity by shining pen light in one eye followed by the other eye (2) extraocular movements by following the pen light up, down, in, out, and laterally	(1) First look at provider's nose, and then hold head still while light is used to look at the eyes (2) While keeping head still, instruct child to use their eyes to follow the light	(1) Pupil does not respond to light (2) Eyes do not follow light equally
V Trigeminal	(1) Test for bilateral facial sensations using a cotton applicator lightly moved from midline laterally on child's forehead, cheeks, and mandible (2) Test muscles of mastication	(1) Respond with yes or no as to whether or not they can feel the sensation of the cotton applicator in each area (2) Open and close mouth	(1) Child reports loss of sensation in an area (2) Deviation while opening or closing mouth could indicate trigeminal nerve dysfunction or possible jaw fracture

Table 3.1 (continued)

Cranial nerve	Type of test	Instruct child to…	When to be concerned
VII Facial	Test for bilateral facial movement	(1) Wrinkle forehead, raise eyebrows, frown, smile, bare teeth, puff out both cheeks (2) Close eyes and keep closed while dentist tries to open them	(1) Asymmetries in facial movement, angle of mouth droops (2) Eyes can be opened with little resistance
VIII Vestibulocochlear	Test hearing by provider facing the child and holding hands adjacent to each of child's ears. The provider then rubs their thumb and index finger of one hand and then switches hands	Point to the ear (right or left) from which the child hears a sound	Unable to hear sound from one ear
IX Glossopharyngeal X Vagus	(1) Intraoral uvula or palate deviation (2) Gag reflex test by stimulating soft palate with cotton applicator (3) Listening to speaking	(1 and 2) Open mouth wide (3) Assess during earlier conversations	(1) Uvula deviates from midline—will deviate toward unaffected side. Palate will move away from affected side (2) No gag response (3) Unable to speak clearly without hoarseness
XI Spinal Accessory	Neck muscle function	Shrug shoulders and rotate head against resistance of provider's hand	Unequal movement and/or strength of the right and left trapezius and sternocleidomastoid muscles
XII Hypoglossal	Tongue movement	Stick out tongue	Tongue deviates from midline—will deviate toward affected side

3.5   Extraoral/Intraoral Examination

The examination process should begin with taking a baseline set of vital signs including temperature, pulse, blood pressure, and respiratory rate, as tolerated by the patient [9]. The patient must undergo a thorough head and neck examination, and this can be done with the child sitting in the dental chair or in an alternate position, e.g., in a knee-to-knee position or with protective stabilization. In a knee-to-knee examination position, the caregiver and dentist sit facing each other with their knees touching. The child sits on the caregiver's lap facing them. The child then lies back into the dentist's lap. While the caregiver holds the child's hands and legs, the dentist can perform an examination (Fig. 3.1).

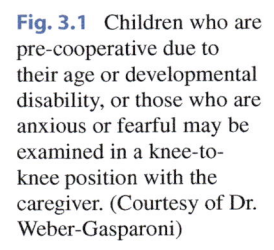

Fig. 3.1 Children who are pre-cooperative due to their age or developmental disability, or those who are anxious or fearful may be examined in a knee-to-knee position with the caregiver. (Courtesy of Dr. Weber-Gasparoni)

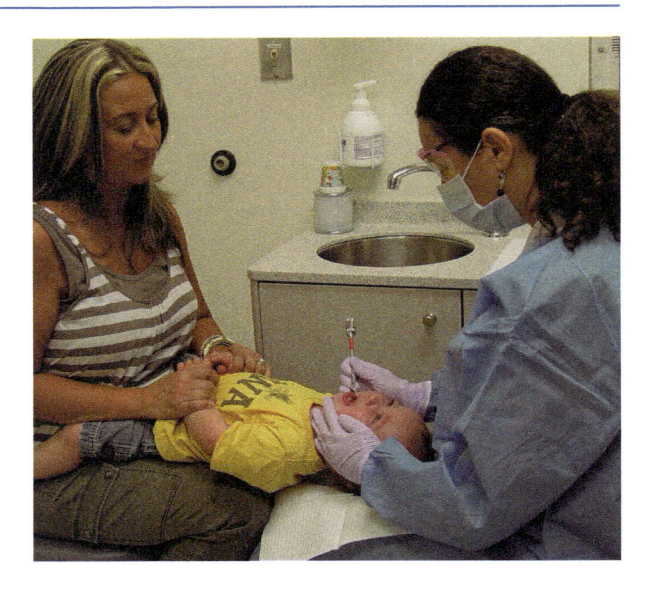

It is important to take photographs of the injuries for documentation.

In order to provide an accurate examination, the head, neck, face, and oral cavity must first be cleaned with water or normal saline. A mild detergent may be used on extraoral soft tissues injuries.

3.5.1 Extraoral Examination

First, examine the face, neck, and lips for lacerations, abrasions, burns, and contusions. The presence of a contusion is most often associated with an underlying bony fracture. The presence of mastoid ecchymosis (Battles sign) is an indication of a fracture of a posterior cranial bone [10]. The presence of orbital hematoma (Raccoon sign) is an indication of an anterior cranial bone fracture [11]. Also, direct injuries to the chin are often associated with condylar fractures. Next, assess for any other signs of bony fractures such as facial asymmetry, an inability to close the mouth, or a deviation in mouth opening. Palpate the bony structure of the face to identify inconsistencies such as a step in the inferior border of the mandible. Additionally, look for cerebral spinal fluid (clear fluid) in the nose, which would also indicate a skull fracture. If bony fractures are suspected obtain an oral and maxillofacial surgery consultation.

3.5.2 Intraoral Examination

Evaluate the intraoral soft tissues for injuries and note all lacerations, abrasions, and contusions. Both sublingual hematomas and vertical lacerations on the alveolus are indicative of an underlying bony fracture. Additional signs of bony fractures include altered occlusion or occlusal interferences not attributed to a displaced tooth (or teeth). Evaluate all of the teeth for any displacement, fracture, mobility, and abnormal response to percussion. Record the direction and distance of each displaced tooth. Assess each fractured tooth and record whether it sustained an uncomplicated or complicated fracture that is limited to the crown or involves the root. Measure the fractured area with relation to the gingival sulcus.

3.6 Radiographic Evaluation

Once the clinical examination is complete, then a radiographic survey of the injured tissues is indicated. A soft tissue radiograph is indicated if there is a penetrating lip wound in order to locate any foreign bodies such as tooth fragments, restorative material, metal, or gravel (Fig. 3.2a, b). To take the radiograph, the film is placed between the lips and the alveolus and the exposure time is reduced to 25% the normal time (Figs. 3.3 and 3.4). If a bony fracture is suspected, panoramic imaging or

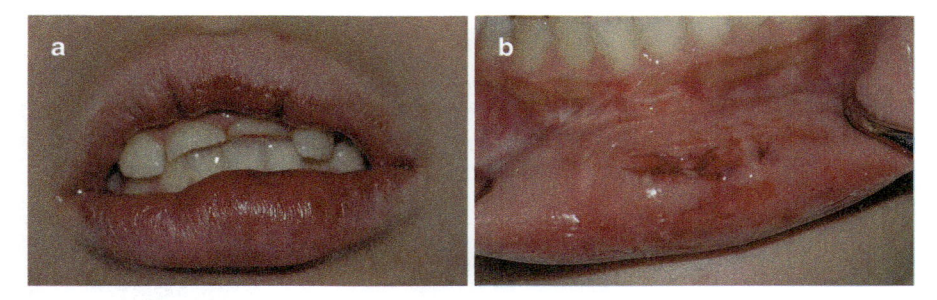

Fig. 3.2 Complicated fracture of maxillary central incisors (**a**) with laceration of the lower lip (**b**). If tooth fragments have not been found at the site of trauma, a soft tissue radiograph is indicated. (Courtesy of Dr. Monica Cipes)

Fig. 3.3 Demonstration of the technique for taking a soft tissue radiograph of the lower lip. The exposure should be reduced to one-fourth of that of tooth structure. (Courtesy of Dr. Ryan Hughes)

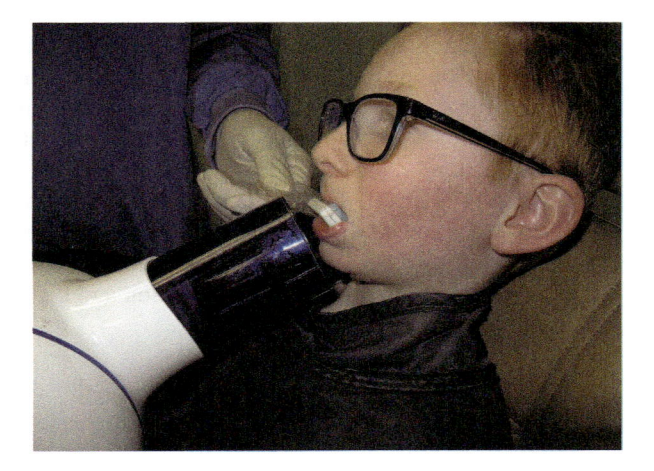

Fig. 3.4 Soft tissue radiograph following fracture of maxillary central incisors. There is no evidence of tooth fragment in the lip. (Courtesy of Dr. Monica Cipes)

Fig. 3.5 Partial image of a panoramic radiograph showing discontinuity of left inferior border of the mandible below the left canine, consistent with a mandibular fracture. (Courtesy of Dr. Mark Engelstad)

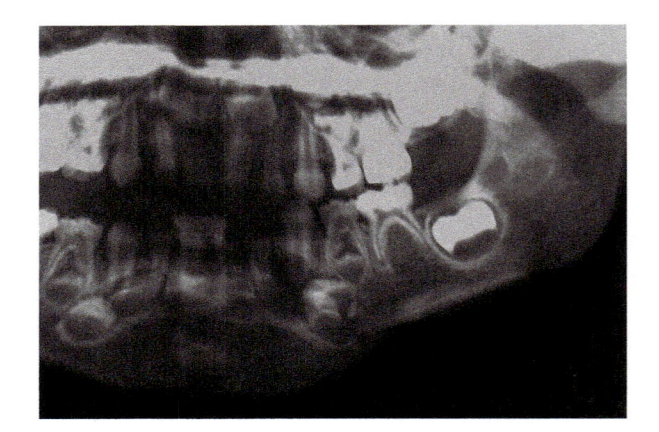

a cone-beam computed tomography may be indicated (Fig. 3.5). Radiographs made of each injured tooth should provide visualization of the apical development, PDL space, periapical pathology, and relationship to developing teeth. Multiple views are required in order to detect displacement of the tooth in its socket as well as the presence of a fractured root [1–3].

If the child is unable to tolerate a radiographic examination even with a caregiver's help, the dentist should consider the advanced behavior management options for the child. It may be best to triage and stabilize the patient for a limited time so that the child may have a thorough evaluation and high quality treatment provided using sedation or general anesthesia.

3.7 Dental Office Preparation

Because pediatric dental traumas present with little to no advanced planning and often outside of regular business hours, it is prudent to have a plan for the office on how emergencies are handled. After-hours on-call coverage is the responsibility of all dental providers for their patients. Established patients should have an after-hours number to call if and when an injury occurs. This number can be forwarded to an office staff member who triages the call or to the dentist directly. The prognosis of an injured tooth depends on the time elapsed between the injury itself and the treatment received. Thus, the dentist should be available to treat his/her patients in a reasonable time or should have previously arranged for an alternate provider to do so.

Additionally, when a patient with a traumatic dental injury arrives at the dental office, it is most efficient to be prepared in advance. A set of trauma treatment supplies should be assembled and ready to use when needed. It may be most convenient to set up a Trauma Kit, a utility box with the necessary supplies inside, and keep it up to date and ready to use when needed (Fig. 3.6).

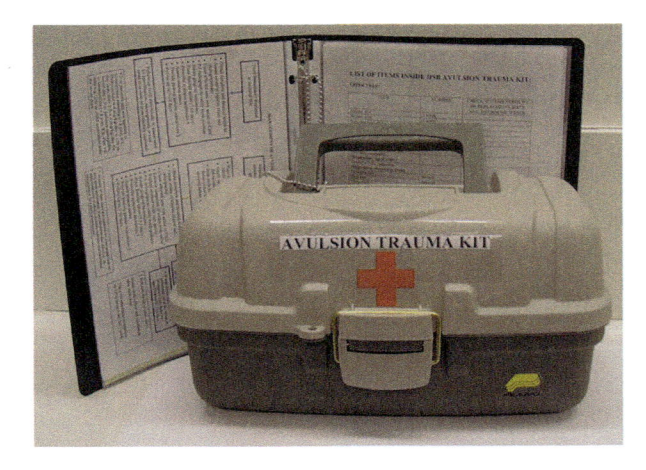

Fig. 3.6 Having a trauma kit prepared in advance and kept up to date increases the likelihood that the dentist will be ready to manage traumatic dental injuries any time of day or night. A notebook containing trauma assessment forms and treatment algorithms also aids in the dentist's preparedness and gives the family confidence that their child will be cared for in a timely way. (Courtesy of Dr. Karin Weber-Gasparoni)

Sample Supplies for the Trauma Kit

Top tray items	Middle tray items	Bottom tray items
Primer/adhesive	Topical anesthetic	End cutter
Blunt needle	Microbrushes	Doxycycline capsules
Composite resin	Calcium hydroxide powder	Composite gun
Fishing line	Empty 2 oz. bottle to mix Doxycycline capsule with 20 mL 0.9% sodium chloride (saline)	Chlorhexidine 0.12%
Flowable composite	Etch Tips	Toothsaver kit
Flowable tips	Local anesthetic carpules	Glass Ionomer
Syringe—5 cc	Cotton applicators	0.9% Sodium chloride saline
Etchant	Sutures	2.0% Neutral sodium fluoride
Arch wires	Smelling salts	Gauze
Cotton rolls		Medicine cups—soak tooth in fluoride

Assessment materials:
- trauma assessment forms
- clipboard
- pen
- penlight
- laminated visual assessment chart with different colored letters
- normal saline

Treatment instruments:
- mirror
- explorer
- scissors
- rubber dam kit
- plastic instrument
- curing light

References

1. Andreasen FM, Andreasen JO. Diagnosis of luxation injuries: the importance of standardized clinical, radiographic and photographic techniques in clinical investigations. Endod Dent Traumatol. 1985;5:160–9.
2. Bakland LK, Andreasen JO. Examination of the dentally traumatized patient. J Calif Dent Assoc. 1996;24:35–44.
3. Andreasen FM, Andreasen JO, Tsukiboshi M, Cohenca N. Examination and diagnosis of dental injuries. In: Andreasen JO, Andreasen FM, Andersson L, editors. Textbook and color atlas of traumatic injuries to the teeth. 5th ed. Hoboken: Wiley-Blackwell; 2019. p. 295–326.
4. Andreasen JO, editor. The dental trauma guide. San Diego: International Association of Dental Traumatology; 2012. https://dentaltraumaguide.org/. Accessed 18 May 2019.

5. American Academy of Pediatric Dentistry. Assessment of acute traumatic injuries. In: Pediatric dentistry reference manual, Vol. 40, No. 6. 2018–2019. http://www.aapd.org/media/Policies_Guidelines/R_AcuteTrauma.pdf. Accessed 18 May 2019.
6. Kopel HM, Johnson R. Examination and neurologic assessment of children with oro-facial trauma. Endod Dent Traumatol. 1985;1:155–9.
7. Glasgow Coma Scale. Institute of Neurological Sciences NHS Greater Glasgow and Clyde. https://www.glasgowcomascale.org/downloads/GCS-Assessment-Aid-English.pdf?v=3. Accessed 18 May 2019.
8. Croll TP, Brooks EB, Schut L, Laurent JP. Rapid neurologic assessment and initial management for the patient with traumatic dental injuries. J Am Dent Assoc. 1980;100:530–4.
9. Davis MJ. Orofacial trauma management. Patient assessment and documentation. N Y State Dent J. 1995;62:93–6.
10. Tubbs RS, Shoja MM, Loukas M, Oakes WJ, Cohen-Gadol A. William Henry Battle and Battle's sign: mastoid ecchymosis as an indicator of basilar skull fracture. J Neurosurg. 2010;112:186–8.
11. Herbella FA, Mudo M, Delmonti C, Braga FM, Del Grande JC. 'Raccoon eyes' (periorbital haematoma) as a sign of skull base fracture. Injury. 2001;32:745–7.

Primary Tooth Crown and Root Fractures

4

In the primary dentition, injuries to the supporting structures (luxation injuries) are more common because the surrounding bone is less dense [1]. An impact is more likely to displace a tooth rather than cause a fracture of the hard tissue. Many retrospective studies of traumatic injuries report that the most common injuries to primary teeth are crown fractures that are limited to the enamel [2, 3]. This is due to the nature of retrospective studies that are looking at visible signs of past trauma. A fracture that is limited to enamel or enamel and dentin is classified as an uncomplicated crown fracture. In the Ellis classification system, it was referred to as a Class I fracture (enamel) or Class II fracture (enamel and dentin). Other types of fractures that affect primary teeth but are less common, are fractures of enamel and dentin with pulp exposure, crown-root fractures, root fractures, and fractures of the alveolus that involve multiple teeth. This chapter focuses on fractures in the primary dentition and discusses treatment, prognosis, and sequelae as well as the behavior guidance techniques that allow safe treatment of the child.

4.1 Uncomplicated Crown Fracture

This type of injury includes fractures of enamel and/or dentin but without a pulp exposure. Currently Ellis Class I and Class II fractures are combined together and referred to as uncomplicated fractures. Fractures limited to enamel may present an esthetic concern and may create a sharp edge that can cause additional trauma to the tongue or soft tissues but are not usually sensitive to air or liquids. When the fracture extends into dentin, sensitivity to temperature is possible.

The evaluation of this type of injury should include a determination of other types of injuries to the same or other teeth. A fall that is significant enough to fracture a tooth may also cause a concussive or luxation injury to one or more teeth. As part of the intraoral and extraoral examination, soft tissue injuries should also be evaluated and addressed.

© Springer Nature Switzerland AG 2020
R. L. Slayton, E. A. Palmer, *Traumatic Dental Injuries in Children*,
https://doi.org/10.1007/978-3-030-25793-4_4

Although the fracture is visible clinically, an intraoral radiograph is indicated to provide a baseline for this tooth and to rule out a root fracture (Fig. 4.1a, b). For very young children, either a periapical radiograph or occlusal radiograph is appropriate. The caregiver should be asked to assist with the radiograph by holding the child on their lap and holding the film or sensor in place once it is positioned by the dentist or dental assistant. If the fractured segment was not found and if there is a laceration of the lip, the dentist should consider a soft tissue radiograph to rule out the possibility of the tooth fragment being imbedded in the lip (Fig. 4.2). In this situation, a radiograph of the lip at one-fourth strength should be made (Fig. 4.3).

4.1.1   Treatment Recommendations

In the primary dentition, treatment is done to address esthetics and discomfort. This may be challenging for the very young child due to their limited ability to cooperate for a procedure that requires good isolation. For enamel only fractures, the sharp

Fig. 4.1 Clinical examination (**a**) and radiographic examination (**b**) show an uncomplicated fracture of the primary left maxillary central incisor with no evidence of luxation or root fracture. (Courtesy of the University of Iowa Department of Pediatric Dentistry)

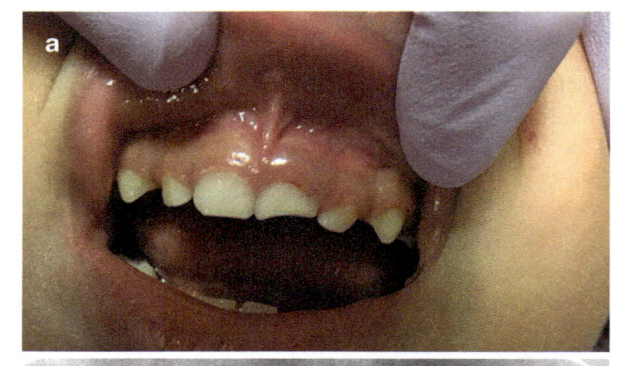
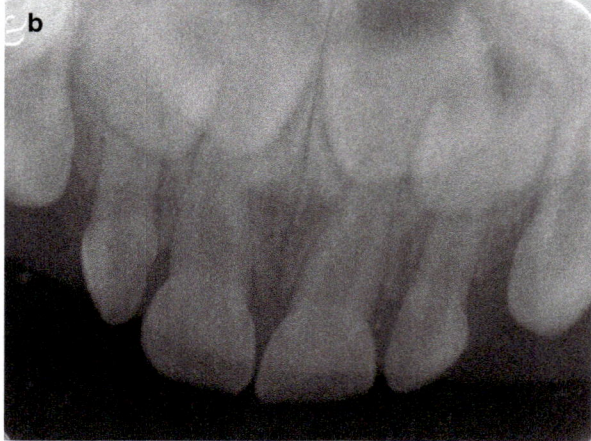

Fig. 4.2 Soft tissue laceration following fracture of maxillary incisors. If tooth fragments were not found at the site of the accident, a soft tissue radiograph is recommended to rule out tooth fragments in the lip. (Courtesy of Dr. Monica Cipes)

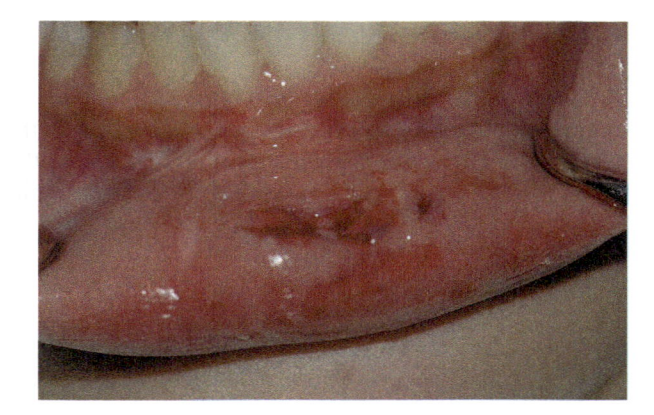

Fig. 4.3 Technique for making a soft tissue radiograph to rule out a tooth fragment in the lip. The exposure should be one-fourth of what is used for the dentition. (Courtesy of Dr. Ryan Hughes)

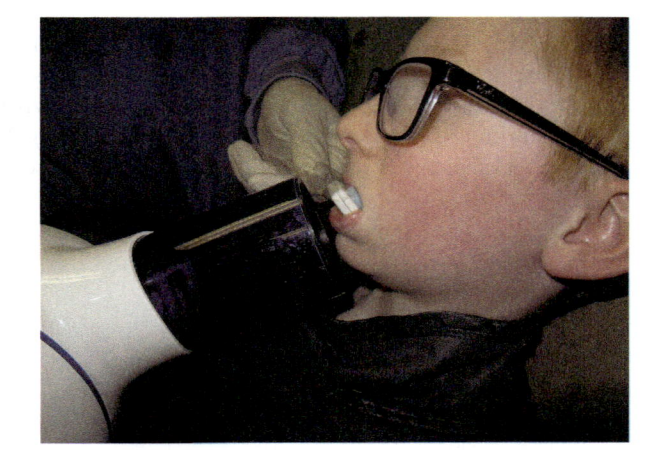

edges should be eliminated to minimize further soft tissue trauma. This can be done using a sand paper disk on a slow speed handpiece. For an enamel-dentin fracture, a restoration can be placed to seal the dentin and prevent microleakage. There is limited evidence to support the need for a restoration when there is a small enamel/dentin fracture as the only injury [4]. The primary goal should be to protect soft tissues from any sharp edges and improve esthetics if the child is able to cooperate for the restorative procedure. A glass ionomer material is recommended due to potential challenges with isolation. If the child will be sedated or under general anesthesia for other treatment, a composite restoration or strip crown can be placed. This type of injury does not require urgent treatment unless the child is in pain or the sharp edges are causing additional soft tissue trauma. In most situations, evaluation can be delayed until normal office hours.

4.1.2 Prognosis

Prognosis for uncomplicated fractures of primary teeth depends on the extent of the injury and the stage of development of the injured tooth. Teeth with an open apex recover from this type of trauma more readily than teeth with a closed apex. There is limited data regarding the prognosis of this type of injury in primary teeth [5].

4.1.3 Sequelae

Even though this is a relatively minor injury, the sequelae may include tooth discoloration, calcific metamorphosis, pulp necrosis, abscess, and/or tooth loss.

4.1.4 Behavior Management

It should be possible to complete a clinical examination for this type of injury for any age child, including those with special health care needs. For very young children, a knee-to-knee exam with a caregiver provides good visibility of the oral cavity. Caregivers are asked to assist with hands and feet during the examination (Fig. 4.4). For older special needs children, it may be helpful to use protective stabilization for

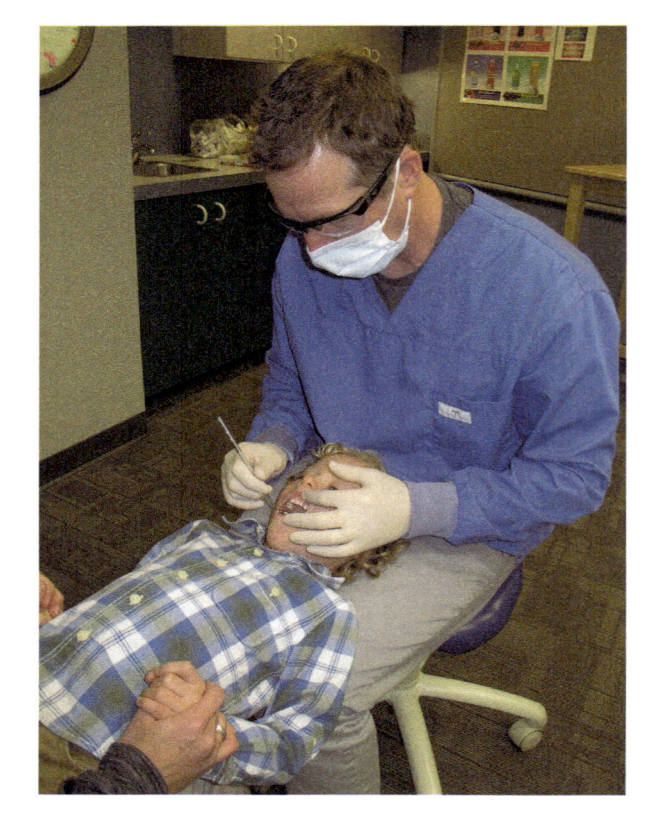

Fig. 4.4 For young or anxious children, a knee-to-knee examination will help the dentist visualize the oral cavity while the caregiver or assistant holds the child's hands and provides reassurance. (Courtesy of Dr. Ryan Hughes)

the clinical examination and radiographs. This was described in more detail in Chaps. 2 and 3.

4.2 Complicated Crown Fracture

A complicated fracture is a fracture of enamel and dentin that exposes the pulp (Fig. 4.5a, b). In the Ellis classification system, this is a Class III injury. The fracture and pulp exposure is apparent clinically. It is a relatively rare injury in the primary dentition with estimates between 0 and 3.2% of traumatized teeth [6]. A radiograph is recommended to rule out root fracture, assess the stage of root development and establish a baseline for future comparison.

4.2.1 Treatment Recommendations

How this type of injury is managed is dictated by the child's behavior, the restorability of the tooth, the child's medical health and time elapsed since the injury. If the child is healthy and cooperative and there is sufficient tooth structure, a direct pulp cap or partial pulpotomy is recommended, followed by a well-sealed restoration. The goal is to maintain the vitality of the pulp until normal exfoliation occurs. If the child is not cooperative, is complex medically, or if the fractured tooth

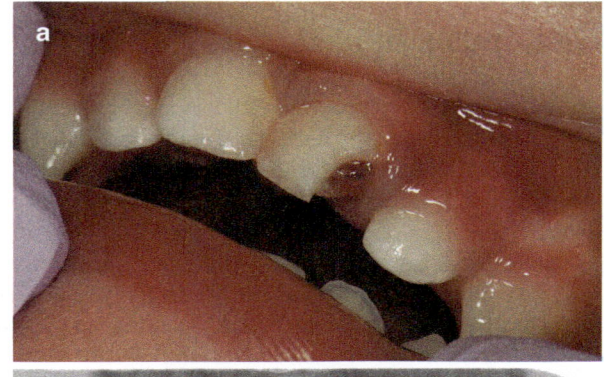
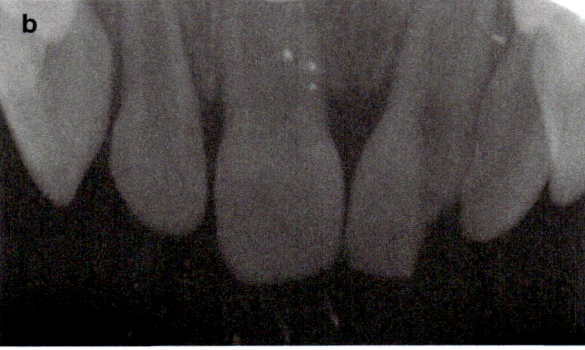

Fig. 4.5 Complicated fracture of primary left maxillary incisor (**a**) with occlusal radiograph (**b**) showing the extent of the fracture. Ideally, the radiograph should show the apex of the incisors to rule out root fracture or luxation. (Courtesy of the University of Iowa Department of Pediatric Dentistry)

is too compromised to restore, extraction is the treatment of choice. In some cases, there is a delay in bringing the child in for evaluation, increasing the chance that the pulp has become necrotic. In this situation, extraction is indicated as soon as possible [7].

Direct pulp cap is accomplished by placing a medicament over the pulp exposure followed by a composite restoration. Recommended medicaments are calcium hydroxide or mineral trioxide aggregate (MTA). If calcium hydroxide is used, a glass ionomer liner should be placed over the calcium hydroxide to form a good seal. This is not needed for MTA [5].

Partial pulpotomy involves providing local anesthesia, rubber dam isolation, and removal of a few millimeters of coronal pulp tissue using a high-speed handpiece with water irrigation. This clearly requires either a cooperative child or the use of sedation or general anesthesia. The medicaments for this procedure are the same as for a direct pulp cap (calcium hydroxide or MTA) and as before, it is crucial that a good seal is made underneath the final restoration.

Extraction may be the best treatment option for the child if it is not possible to obtain good isolation due to behavior. This is still a challenging option because it is necessary to anesthetize the tooth and to perform the extraction in a safe and compassionate manner. In an office setting, especially after-hours, sedation may not be a safe option. In this case, other types of advanced behavior guidance such as nitrous oxide, protective stabilization or restraint by the caregiver may be necessary. In a hospital emergency room, there are often more options for pharmacologic management in collaboration with the medical team.

4.2.2   Follow-Up

If a restoration was placed, the child should be seen for a follow-up clinical exam in 1 week to make sure the restoration is intact and to document that healing is taking place. Additional clinical and radiographic examinations should be done at 6–8 weeks and at 1 year [5]. Positive findings include vital pulp, continued root development, and no sign of periapical pathology. Discoloration and/or evidence of calcific metamorphosis may occur and does not necessarily indicate treatment failure. Negative findings such as periapical pathology or abscess would indicate that treatment has failed and the tooth should be extracted (Fig. 4.6).

4.2.3   Prognosis

The most frequent treatment option for this type of injury is extraction. There is limited data regarding the prognosis for complicated fractures in primary teeth that are treated with direct pulp cap or partial pulpotomy. Case-based literature has documented the success of partial pulpotomy using calcium hydroxide [6]. In this case study, follow-up at 21 weeks demonstrated continued root development and the formation of a dentin bridge at the site of the exposure. In a second case reported by

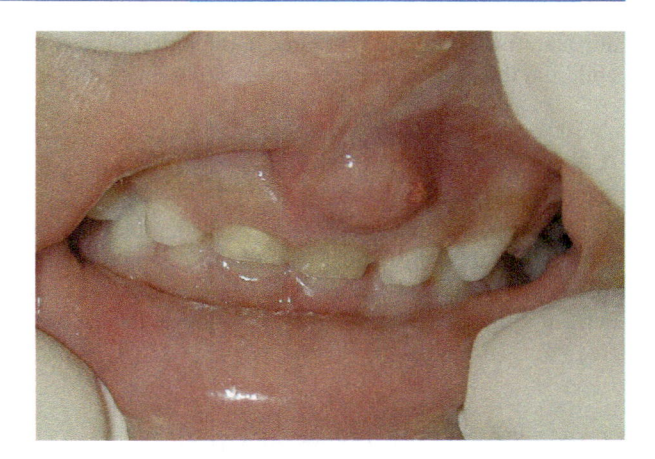

Fig. 4.6 The primary left maxillary incisor is discolored with evidence of a parulis indicating presence of an abscess. A radiograph is indicated to confirm the diagnosis and to assess the adjacent teeth. Extraction of the abscessed tooth is indicated

Kupietsky and Holan, a similar partial pulpotomy was performed and the tooth remained vital at the 2-year follow-up visit [8]. These authors assert the importance of maintaining the traumatized primary tooth when possible. This is more likely to be successful when the child is seen as soon after the trauma as possible.

4.2.4 Sequelae

Discoloration and/or evidence of calcific metamorphosis may occur and does not necessarily indicate treatment failure. Premature extraction of primary teeth may significantly delay the eruption of the permanent successor. Failed treatment resulting in periapical pathology can have negative consequences for the permanent successor, including developmental defects of enamel, delayed eruption, enhanced eruption, or ectopic eruption [7, 9].

4.2.5 Behavior Management

Initial examination of a child with a complicated crown fracture can be accomplished in the traditional clinic setting either in the dental chair or in a knee-to-knee position with the caregiver. If extraction is the treatment of choice, and there are no medical contraindications, the tooth or teeth can be extracted using a combination of non-pharmaologic and pharmacologic techniques. Extreme care should be taken to ensure adequate local anesthesia has been provided and to protect the airway from inadvertent aspiration of the tooth as it is removed. This can be accomplished by using a 2 × 2 gauze shield held in place behind the maxillary incisors and draped over the tongue and throat. Since extraction of a primary tooth is a relatively quick procedure, it can be accomplished with limited cooperation from the child.

If the tooth is to be retained through the use of a direct pulp cap or partial pulpotomy, the behavior needs to be cooperative enough so that local anesthesia, adequate isolation, pulp therapy, and restoration can be performed. In very young children, this may require the use of sedation as described in Chap. 2.

4.3 Crown/Root Fracture

This type of fracture involves enamel, dentin, and root structure with or without exposure of the pulp. This type of injury is rare in the primary dentition. The fractured tooth fragment that extends subgingivally may be very loose. It is normally evident clinically. A radiograph is made to determine the position and number of fragments (Fig. 4.7a, b).

4.3.1 Treatment Recommendations

Treatment is dictated by the severity of the injury, the size of the loose fragment, exposure of pulp, the behavior of the child, medical diagnosis, and time elapsed since the injury. If the fragment is small and the remaining tooth is stable with no

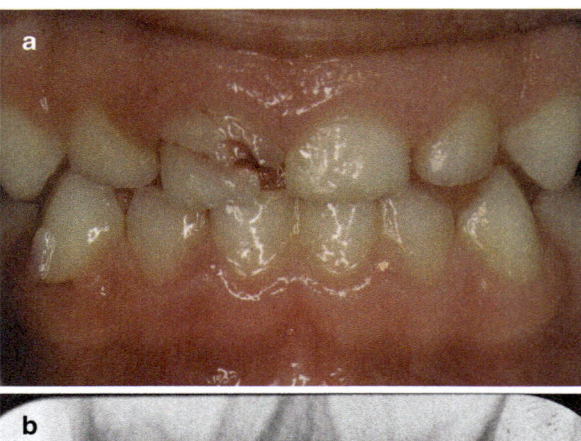
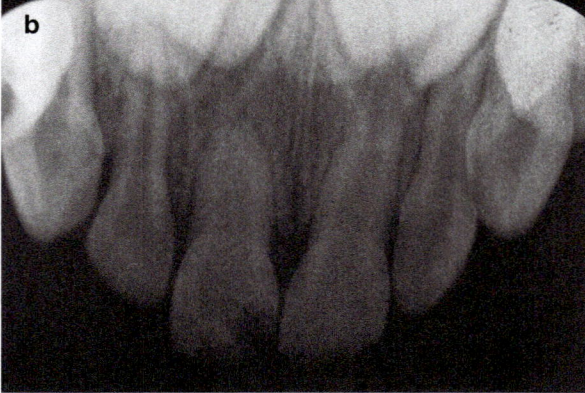

Fig. 4.7 Crown/root fracture of primary incisor with pulp exposure. Clinical (**a**) and radiographic (**b**) evaluation indicates that extraction is the best option. (Courtesy of Dr. Simon Jenn-Yih Lin)

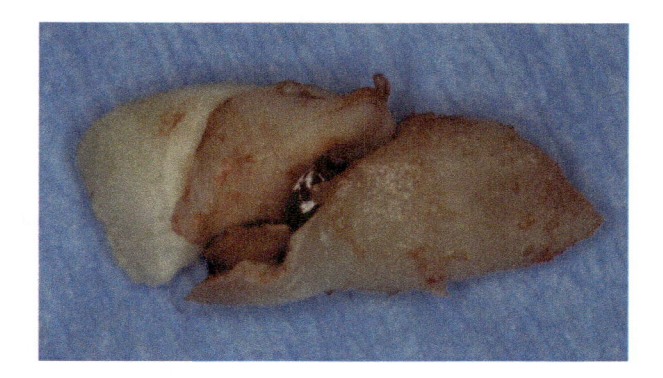

Fig. 4.8 Extracted tooth with crown/root fracture. In this case, extraction was the only option as the fracture line extended well beyond the gingival margin. (Courtesy of Dr. Simon Jenn-Yih Lin)

pulp exposure, removal of the fractured tooth fragment and restoration of the remaining coronal segment is indicated. If removal of the fragment reveals a pulp exposure, either a direct pulp cap or partial pulpotomy is performed using calcium hydroxide, followed by a well-sealed restoration. The final option is extraction of the fragment and remaining tooth [1]. This type of injury is likely to be symptomatic because the loose fragment will be disrupted during eating or drinking. It is possible that there is a delay in seeking treatment and this will influence treatment decisions because the tooth may have become non-vital prior to coming to the office for care. If this is the case, extraction is the best option (Fig. 4.8).

4.3.2 Follow-Up

If the fragment is removed and the tooth retained, the patient should be seen for a clinical examination in 1 week and then clinical and radiographic examinations in 6–8 weeks, 1 year, and every year afterwards until the tooth exfoliates [5]. If the pulp was exposed and a pulpotomy was performed followed by a restoration, a similar series of follow-up examinations are indicated.

4.3.3 Prognosis

The prognosis of a crown-root fracture in primary teeth depends on the severity and extent of the injury. If the tooth is maintained, the prognosis is improved if there was no pulp exposure and if the restoration provides a good seal and remains intact. Subsequent trauma to the same tooth or teeth decreases the prognosis. In a study of traumatic dental injuries to the primary dentition, Mendoza-Mendoza et al. [10] followed 17 patients with crown-root fractures and found no complication in any of the 16 patients that presented for follow-up. In a case study of 28 primary teeth with crown-root fracture, 31% of the teeth were treated with pulpectomy and the remaining teeth were either partially or completely extracted. The patients were followed until eruption of the permanent successors and no complications were reported [11].

These studies demonstrate that the evidence available for this type of injury in primary teeth and outcomes of treatment are limited.

4.3.4 Sequelae

Sequelae are similar to the primary tooth fractures described previously. Discoloration and/or evidence of calcific metamorphosis may occur and does not necessarily indicate treatment failure. Failed treatment resulting in periapical pathology can have negative consequences for the permanent successor, including developmental defects of enamel, delayed eruption, enhanced eruption, or ectopic eruption [7, 9]. If the injury results primarily in a fracture, without displacement, the risk of damage to the developing tooth is minimal. If the tooth is extracted, it may cause delay of eruption of the permanent successor.

4.3.5 Behavior Management

For a crown-root fracture of a primary tooth, deferring treatment is not a reasonable option because it will most likely be symptomatic. All of the treatment options require local anesthesia and some level of intervention that relies on cooperation from the patient.

Initial examination of a child with a complicated crown fracture can be accomplished in the traditional clinic setting either in the dental chair or in a knee-to-knee position with the caregiver. If extraction is the treatment of choice, and there are no medical contraindications, the tooth or teeth can be extracted using a combination of non-pharmacologic and pharmacologic techniques. Extreme care should be taken to ensure adequate local anesthesia has been provided and to protect the airway from inadvertent aspiration of the tooth fragments as they are removed. This can be accomplished by using a 2×2 gauze shield held in place behind the maxillary incisors and draped over the tongue and throat. Since extraction of a primary tooth is a relatively quick procedure, it can be accomplished with limited cooperation from the child.

If the tooth is to be restored or if there is a need for a direct pulp cap or partial pulpotomy, the behavior needs to be cooperative enough so that local anesthesia, adequate isolation, pulp therapy, and restoration can be performed. In very young children, this may require the use of sedation as described in Chap. 2.

4.4 Root Fracture

Root fractures in primary teeth are relatively rare. In a study of root fractures in an Italian Emergency Center, Marjorana et al. reported a prevalence of 3.8% among a sample of 480 primary tooth injuries [12]. This injury is described by the location along the length of the root. It may be in the apical third, mid-third, or coronal third.

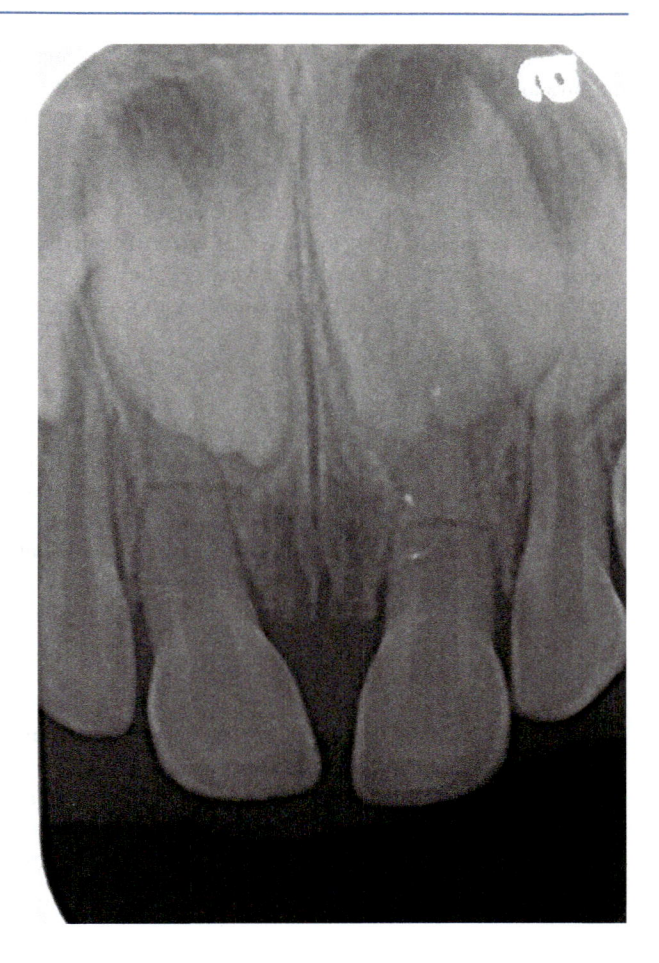

Fig. 4.9 Root fractures are evident in the apical third of the right primary maxillary incisor and in the middle third of the left primary maxillary incisor. In this case, the fracture lines were evident in a single periapical radiograph. (Courtesy of Dr. Dennis J. McTigue)

Root fractures in the cervical third have the poorest prognosis and the most mobility. Diagnosis is made radiographically and may require two or three images with different angles. The coronal segment may or may not be displaced (Fig. 4.9).

4.4.1 Treatment Recommendations

No treatment is needed if the fracture is in the middle or apical third of the root and if the coronal segment is not displaced [1, 5]. If the fracture is in the coronal third, if the segment is displaced or if there is more than physiologic mobility of the segment, it should be extracted. If extraction of the coronal segment is done, the remaining apical segment should be left in place rather than attempting to remove it. In most cases, the remaining root fragment will resorb as the permanent tooth erupts [5].

Splinting is considered an option when the coronal fragment is displaced and mobile and the child is cooperative enough to tolerate this treatment. In a study of 10 patients with 16 root fractures, the most common location was mid-root [13]. Repositioning was done if needed and then the teeth were splinted with an orthodontic wire for 4–8 weeks. During the period of the study, no teeth required pulp therapy, the root fragments were resorbed, and permanent successors erupted in the expected manner without evidence of enamel defects [13]. The primary goal of a splint is to minimize sensitivity during function, not to stimulate repair of the fractured segment, as is done in permanent tooth root fractures [7].

4.4.2 Follow-Up

If there is no displacement and the tooth is retained, the child should be seen for a clinical examination in 1 week and then a clinical and radiographic exam in 6–8 weeks, in 1 year, and every year until exfoliation [5]. If the tooth is extracted, clinical and radiographic examinations should be done on an annual basis to monitor resorption of the remaining root fragment and eruption of the permanent successor.

4.4.3 Prognosis

It is unlikely that the two fragments will be repaired over time. Case studies have demonstrated that the apical fragment will be resorbed as the permanent successor erupts [13]. Depending on the degree of displacement and the location of the fracture, it is possible that the pulp will become inflamed or necrotic. There is limited data regarding outcomes for primary tooth root fractures and this reinforces the need for consistency in diagnosis and outcomes reporting.

4.4.4 Sequelae

Among cases reported in the IADT Trauma Guide, 9.4% of teeth with root fracture had pulp necrosis and 9.2% had pulp obliteration after 1 year [14]. If the tooth was not displaced, it is unlikely that there will be sequelae to the permanent successor.

4.4.5 Behavior Management

Cooperation is needed for the clinical examination and radiographs and this can be accomplished using non-pharmacologic methods with the help of a caregiver. In most cases, no treatment is recommended. However, if the tooth has been displaced or is mobile and the treatment decision is to place a splint or extract the tooth, then additional, more advanced behavior guidance methods may be required as described above and in Chap. 2.

4.5 Fractures of the Alveolar Process

A fracture of the alveolar process in a young child is a severe injury with complicated management considerations. It is usually caused by a forceful impact directed perpendicular to the mandible or maxilla. It may also be caused by the child falling on an object such as a toy. Multiple teeth involved in the injury move together as a unit when mobility is evaluated. This injury usually results in displacement of teeth resulting in occlusal interference [1]. In some situations, a vertical line in the gingiva is visible on either side of the fractured segment (Fig. 4.10). The diagnosis is usually evident from clinical findings but one or more radiographs are indicated to thoroughly evaluate the extent of the injury. It may be helpful to make a lateral radiograph to assess the relationship between the primary tooth roots and the developing permanent teeth.

4.5.1 Treatment Recommendations

The soft tissue in the area of the injury should be irrigated with saline or chlorhexidine to remove any debris. The fractured, displaced segment is repositioned and splinted using a semirigid splint. Splinting materials should be readily available and can consist of bonded resin or orthodontic wire. The splint should stay in place for 3–4 weeks. In very young children, there may not be adequate numbers of erupted teeth to use as anchorage for the mobile segment. In this case, repositioning and a strict adherence to a soft or liquid diet should be recommended. Teeth should be maintained while bone is healing. If extraction becomes necessary, it should be done at a later time. Young children may require treatment under sedation or general anesthesia.

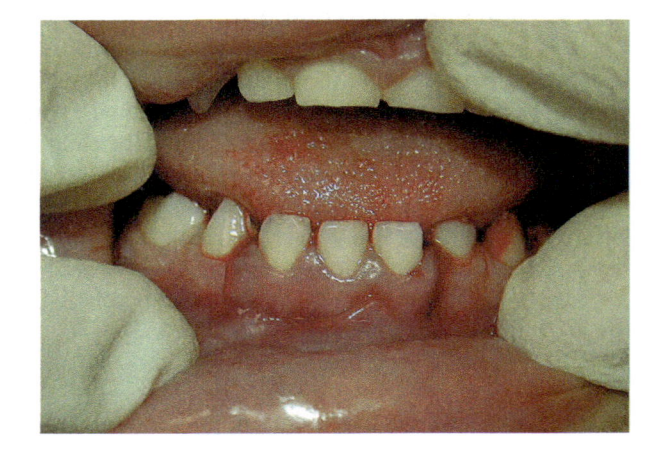

Fig. 4.10 An alveolar fracture in the primary dentition may often present with vertical lines on either side of the segment that is fractured. All three teeth move as one when mobility is tested

4.5.2 Follow-Up

The child should be seen for a clinical examination at 1 week. At 3–4 weeks, the splint is removed and a clinical and radiographic examination is performed. The child should be seen for clinical and radiographic examination after 6–8 week, 1 year, and every year until the teeth exfoliate [5].

4.5.3 Prognosis

In a series of 26 teeth from 10 patients, the most common outcomes were pulp obliteration (38.5%), tooth loss (23.1%), and pulp necrosis (15.4%) [14]. There are limited reports of alveolar fracture in the primary dentition. In one case study of a 5-year-old boy, Akin et al. [15] reported that after following the IADT Guidelines, there was a favorable outcome for the alveolar fracture and the affected primary teeth and there was no evidence of negative sequelae for the permanent teeth [15].

4.5.4 Sequelae

Long-term studies of outcomes related to alveolar fractures in the primary dentition are very limited. The sequelae are dictated by the severity of the injury, time delay in receiving care, treatment provided, and age at the time of injury. Teeth in the displaced segment may require root canal treatment or extraction once the alveolar bone has healed. For injuries that result in palatal or lingual displacement of the segment, the developing permanent tooth is not likely to be damaged as part of the traumatic injury but is at risk of trauma when the segment is repositioned and splinted. Permanent teeth are at risk for enamel defects.

4.5.5 Behavior Management

Cooperation is needed for the clinical examination and radiographs and this can be accomplished using non-pharmacologic methods with the help of a caregiver. Because of the severity of this type of injury, the child is likely to be directed to the hospital emergency department for evaluation and treatment. Many small, community hospitals don't have dentists on staff, so the child will most likely need to be referred to a tertiary care center. Unfortunately, this causes a delay in treatment. Also, because the repositioning and splinting of a displaced segment of teeth and alveolar bone requires good anesthesia and isolation, this type of injury is best treated under general anesthesia.

4.6 Patient Instructions

The patient should be advised to eat soft foods or liquids for 10–14 days. They should avoid biting or tearing food with their injured teeth for up to 6 weeks. After the first 2 weeks, they may eat more solid foods if it is cut into small pieces. If the child is using a sippy cup, care should be taken so that they aren't putting undue pressure on the front teeth when drinking from the cup. It may be preferable to use a cup without a lid.

Non-nutritive sucking habits create a challenge for healing after trauma to anterior teeth. The habit is usually soothing for the child but increases the risk for additional trauma to the teeth or alveolus. Pacifier use should be restricted or eliminated during the healing process.

Good oral hygiene following a traumatic dental injury is essential for good healing. The teeth and oral tissues are likely to be sensitive, so a soft toothbrush should be used after each meal to remove food debris and plaque. The bristles can be further softened by running the brush under warm water before use. Alcohol free chlorhexidine (0.12%) should be applied to the teeth in the area of the trauma using a soft brush or cotton swab. Older children who are able to rinse and spit should swish with chlorhexidine 2–3 times per day. This will minimize the plaque buildup in the area of trauma.

For very young children, it is important to prevent a second injury while the first injury is still healing. This will seriously decrease the prognosis of the injured teeth. For older children who are involved in sports activities, it is best to avoid these activities for 2–3 weeks and then wear a protective mouthguard once the sporting activity has begun again.

Advice about possible complications and future sequelae should be provided to the caregiver. It may be beneficial to have this information in written form that the family can take home and refer to at a later time. It can also be available on the clinic's website. The signs to watch for during the first few weeks include swelling, increased mobility, infection, or drainage from a fistula. Evidence of increased redness or infection should be a sign to return to the office for evaluation. Bleeding should be under control by the time the child leaves the office but if bleeding continues or starts again after returning home, the family should contact the office. As healing progresses, the caregivers may notice a change in the color of injured teeth (gray or yellow), swelling, abscess formation, increased mobility of the tooth, and/ or detachment of the splint (if present).

Children may or may not complain of pain. If pain is keeping the child awake at night or interfering with their ability to eat or drink, they should be given the appropriate dose of liquid ibuprofen or acetaminophen to keep them comfortable.

It is important to inform caregivers about any possible complications that may affect the permanent teeth. This should also be explained as part of the written documentation given at the time of dismissal.

References

1. Flores MT, Holan G, Andreasen JO, Lauridsen E. Injuries to the primary dentition. In: Andreasen JO, Andreasen FM, Andersson L, editors. Textbook and color atlas of traumatic injuries to the teeth. 5th ed. Hoboken: Wiley-Blackwell; 2019. p. 556–88.
2. Jorge KO, Moyses SJ, Ferreira e Ferreira E, Ramos-Jorge ML, de Araujo Zarzar PM. Prevalence and factors associated to dental trauma in infants 1-3 years of age. Dent Traumatol. 2009;25:185–9.

3. Viegas CM, Scarpelli AC, Carvalho AC, Ferreira FM, Pordeus IA, Paiva SM. Predisposing factors for traumatic dental injuries in Brazilian preschool children. Eur J Paediatr Dent. 2010;11:59–65.
4. Ravn JJ. Follow-up study of permanent incisors with enamel-dentin fractures after acute trauma. Scand J Dent Res. 1981;89:355–65.
5. Malmgren B, Adreasen JO, Flores MT, Robertson A, DiAngelis AJ, Andersson L, Cavalleri G, Cohenca N, Day P, Hicks ML, Malmgren O, Moule AJ, Onetto J, Tsukiboshi M, International Association of Dental Traumatology. International Association of Dental Traumatology Guidelines for the management of traumatic dental injuries: 3. Injuries in the primary dentition. Dent Traumatol. 2012;28:174–82.
6. Ram D, Holan G. Partial pulpotomy in a traumatized primary incisor with pulp exposure: case report. Pediatr Dent. 1994;16:46–8.
7. Holan G, McTigue DJ. Introduction to dental trauma: managing traumatic injuries in the primary dentition. In: Nowak AJ, Christensen JR, Mabry TR, Townsend JA, Wells MH, editors. Pediatric dentistry infancy through adolescence. Philadelphia: Elsevier; 2019. p. 227–43.
8. Kupietzky A, Holan G. Treatment of crown fractures with pulp exposure in primary incisors. Pediatr Dent. 2003;25:241–7.
9. Andreasen JO, Flores MT, Lauridsen E. Injuries to developing teeth. In: Andreasen JO, Andreasen FM, Andersson L, editors. Textbook and color atlas of traumatic injuries to the teeth. 5th ed. Hoboken: Wiley-Blackwell; 2019. p. 589–625.
10. Mendoza-Mendoza A, Iglesias-Linares A, Yanez-Vico RM, Abalos-Labruzzi C. Prevalence and complications of trauma to the primary dentition in a subpopulation of Spanish children in southern Europe. Dent Traumatol. 2015;31:144–9.
11. Costa VP, Oliveira LJ, Rosa DP, Cademartori MG, Torriani DD. Crown-root fractures in primary teeth: a case series study of 28 cases. Braz Dent J. 2016;27:234–8.
12. Majorana A, Pasini S, Bardellini E, Keller E. Clinical and epidemiological study of traumatic root fractures. Dent Traumatol. 2002;18:77–80.
13. Kim G-T, Sohn M, Ahn HJ, Lee D-W, Choi SC. Intra-alveolar root fracture in primary teeth. Pediatr Dent. 2012;34:e215–8.
14. Andreasen JO, editor. The dental trauma guide. San Diego: International Association of Dental Traumatology; 2012. https://dentaltraumaguide.org/. Accessed 1/3/2019.
15. Akin A, Uysal S, Cehreli ZC. Segmental alveolar process fracture involving primary incisors: treatment and 24-month follow up. Dent Traumatol. 2011;27:63–6.

Primary Tooth Luxation Injuries

5

Luxation injuries occur when teeth are displaced out of the socket as a result of a traumatic injury. When children fall, teeth are more likely to be displaced than fractured because the supporting bone is less dense than in the permanent dentition [1]. The direction of the displacement and severity of the injury will influence the risk of injury to the developing permanent teeth. This chapter will discuss each type of luxation injury, how they should be managed, the prognosis and sequelae that are likely, and what behavior guidance techniques may need to be used to provide safe treatment.

5.1 Concussion and Subluxation

A concussive injury to one or more teeth does not result in displacement or fracture. There may be bleeding around the sulcus of the tooth and it may be sensitive to touch (Fig. 5.1). Diagnosis is made from clinical findings and description of the injury. Subluxation results in loosening of the tooth without displacement. Even a few days after the injury, mild mobility may be detected. An intraoral radiograph should be made to rule out root fracture and to establish a baseline. Frequently, a caregiver is not aware of this trauma unless they witnessed the child falling or noticed bleeding around the base of the tooth at the time of the injury.

5.1.1 Treatment Recommendations

No treatment is needed and the prognosis for teeth with this type of injury is good. In many cases, the caregivers report this injury over the phone, or it is mentioned at a regular check-up appointment. The most important instructions are for the caregiver to maintain good oral hygiene and to have the child eat a soft diet for a few days. A prescription for chlorhexidine 0.12% is recommended to assist with

© Springer Nature Switzerland AG 2020
R. L. Slayton, E. A. Palmer, *Traumatic Dental Injuries in Children*,
https://doi.org/10.1007/978-3-030-25793-4_5

managing plaque buildup around the injured teeth. This can either be brushed, applied with a cotton swab or for older children, swished in the mouth and expectorated.

5.1.2 Follow-Up

The International Association of Dental Traumatology (IADT) Guidelines recommend a clinical examination at 1 week and at 6–8 weeks [2]. Evaluation of discolored teeth should be done on at least an annual basis.

5.1.3 Prognosis

The tooth may become discolored (yellow or gray) (Fig. 5.2). Discoloration warrants clinical and radiographic evaluation to determine if the tooth is necrotic. One

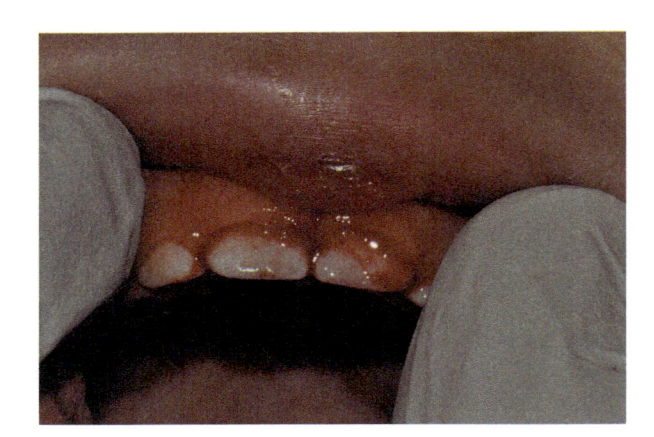

Fig. 5.1 Subluxation injury to primary maxillary incisors. Clinical findings include bleeding around the sulcus and mild mobility. (Courtesy of Dr. Simon Jenn-Yih Lin)

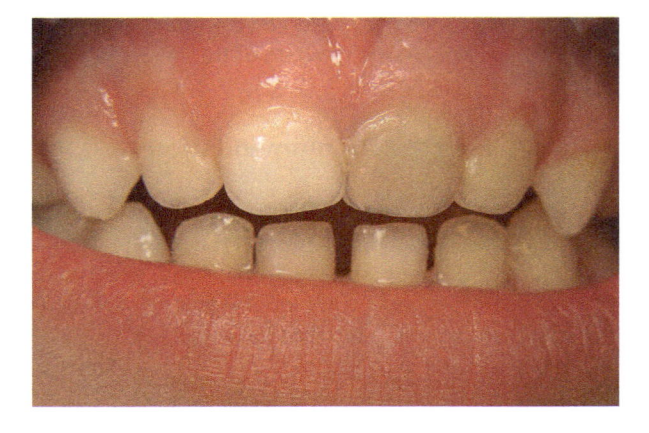

Fig. 5.2 Discolored primary incisor after traumatic injury. (Courtesy of Dr. Travis Nelson)

study of discolored primary incisors following trauma found that there is a fivefold increase in these teeth being necrotic compared to non-discolored traumatized incisors [3]. In a prospective study of discolored traumatized primary incisors, Holan reported that in 52% of teeth, the color faded or became yellowish while 48% remained dark [4]. More than 50% of the teeth that remained dark were asymptomatic until their normal exfoliation. It is clear from these studies that both clinical and radiographic findings are essential for evaluating teeth after trauma and making appropriate treatment decisions.

There are a few reports of complications following subluxation injuries. Some of these were due to delays in treatment, making it difficult to verify the original diagnosis [1]. In one study of 96 subluxated teeth that were followed regularly, 13 teeth developed necrosis of the pulp and 11 teeth displayed root resorption [5]. In a retrospective study of children with concussion or subluxation dental injuries, Lauridsen et al. reported an 8.6% risk for pulp canal obliteration, 5.7% risk for pulp necrosis, and 5.6% risk for tooth loss among children with injuries diagnosed as concussions [6]. For subluxation injuries, the risk of pulp canal obliteration was 23.2%, pulp necrosis was 8.3%, infection-related resorption was 2.6%, and tooth loss was 8.5% [6]. No teeth were ankylosed and the majority of complications were diagnosed within the first year after the injury. No treatment was provided at the time of injury, as indicated by the IADT Guidelines [2].

5.1.4 Sequelae

If the injury was limited to concussion of one or more primary teeth, the risk for pulpal or periodontal complications is low. As noted above, the risk for pulp necrosis is slightly higher with subluxation injuries, but still relatively low. It is unlikely that there will be any sequelae affecting the developing permanent successors when the injury is limited to concussion or subluxation injuries.

5.1.5 Behavior Guidance

It should be possible to complete a clinical examination for this type of injury for any age child, including those with special health care needs. For very young children, a knee-to-knee exam with a caregiver provides good visibility of the oral cavity. Caregivers are asked to assist with hands and feet during the examination. Caregivers may need to help with X-rays.

5.2 Lateral Luxation

Traumatic dental injury that results in the displacement of the tooth either palatally or labially is described as a lateral luxation. It may result in occlusal interference and therefore, needs to be managed in a timely way (Fig. 5.3a). An intraoral

Fig. 5.3 Lateral luxation of primary incisors resulting in occlusal interference (**a**). In the occlusal radiograph (**b**), the roots appear shortened due to the palatal position of the crowns. Extraction is indicated

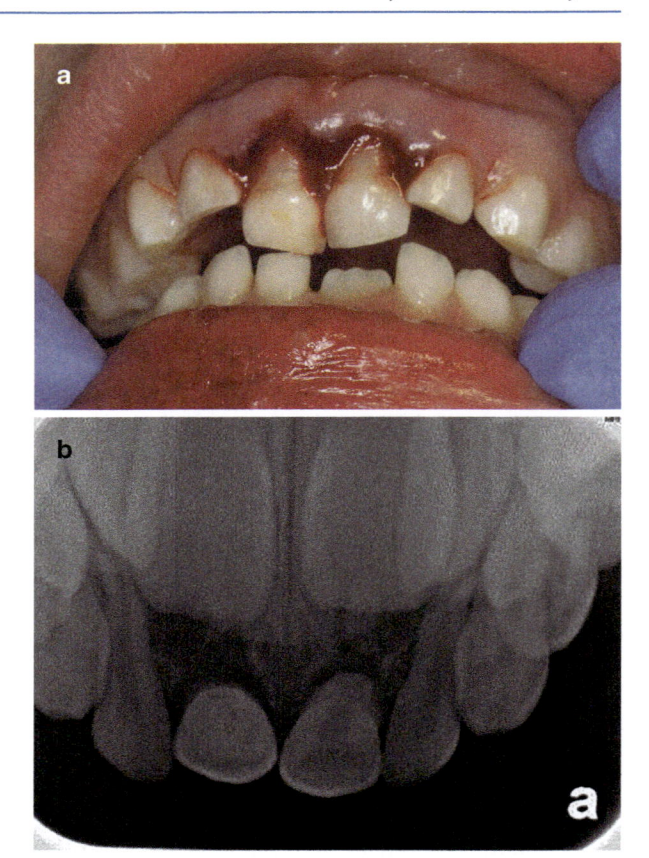

occlusal radiograph is indicated to rule out a root fracture and to establish baseline (Fig. 5.3b). Teeth that are luxated with the crown positioned labially are at a much greater risk of causing damage to the developing permanent teeth (Fig. 5.4). When teeth are luxated palatally or lingually, there is a greater risk of perforation of the root through the buccal plate of bone. Diagnosis of this type of injury is evident clinically because the tooth or teeth are out of alignment with other teeth in the arch. An occlusal radiograph should be made to evaluate the position of the primary tooth root relative to the permanent successor.

5.2.1 Treatment Recommendations

Treatment is dictated by the extent of the injury, time since the injury occurred, position of the root relative to the permanent successor, medical diagnosis, and behavior of the child. With minor displacement and no occlusal interference, it is recommended to allow the tooth to reposition spontaneously [2]. If there is occlusal interference, repositioning is indicated. This necessitates the use of local anesthesia.

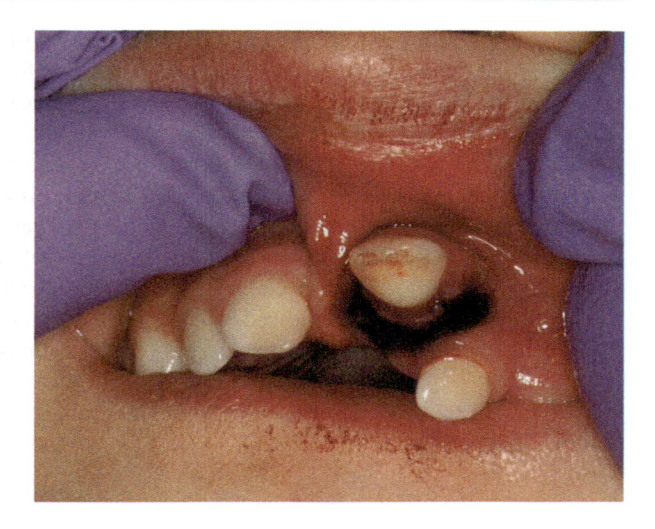

Fig. 5.4 Labial luxation of primary left maxillary central incisor with fracture of alveolar bone. A labial luxation of the crown increases the risk of injury to the developing permanent incisor as does the fracture of the alveolus. Extraction is indicated. (Courtesy of Dr. Simon Jenn-Yih Lin)

When the tooth is displaced palatally, the root apex may have broken through the buccal bone and will require slight extrusive pressure before repositioning it in the socket. With severe luxation, extraction may be the best option.

5.2.2   Follow-Up

It is important to monitor the vitality of the primary tooth, the continued root development and the eruption path of the permanent successor. In young children, it is often difficult to obtain an accurate pulp vitality test and the dentist must rely on clinical findings such as radiographic findings. A clinical exam should be completed at 1 week and at 2–3 weeks. Subsequently, both a clinical and radiographic examination should be done at 6–8 weeks and 1 year [2].

5.2.3   Prognosis

The severity of the injury and how quickly the tooth is repositioned are key factors affecting the prognosis of the primary tooth. It should be monitored regularly to assess vitality. It is likely that primary teeth with lateral luxation will be extracted to avoid additional trauma to the developing permanent tooth. Pulp necrosis and tooth discoloration related to pulpal obliteration are common. There are a few studies that have reported on complications related to lateral luxation injuries in primary teeth. Lauridsen et al. reported on the risk for pulp necrosis (PN), pulp canal obliteration (PCO), infection-related resorption (IRR), ankylosis-related resorption (ARR), and premature tooth loss (PTL) in 331 primary teeth with lateral luxation that were evaluated on a regular basis until exfoliation of the primary tooth [7]. The authors found that 95% of the teeth realigned spontaneously within 1 year. The most common complication was pulp canal obliteration (41.3%) followed by premature tooth loss (24.8%) and pulp necrosis (19.8%) [7]. In a separate study by Soporowski et al., the authors reported on 80 primary teeth with lateral luxation that were either repositioned or observed [8]. Pulp necrosis was seen in 50% of the teeth that were repositioned compared to 17% of the teeth that were observed. Ankylosis occurred in approximately 7% of both groups and calcific changes occurred more frequently in the observation group (15.4%) than in the teeth that were repositioned (3.6%). Data from the IADT Trauma Guide shows the most common finding to be pulp canal obliteration (41.3%) followed by tooth loss (28.3%) and pulp necrosis (18.8%) [9]. There was a very low risk of ankylosis (1.4%) in this database.

5.2.4 Sequelae

Sequelae for the primary tooth include pulp necrosis, calcific metamorphosis, premature tooth loss, and inflammatory root resorption. For the permanent tooth, there is a risk of enamel defects such as opacity or enamel hypoplasia, particularly if the tooth is luxated labially, causing the root to contact the developing permanent tooth crown. Other possible sequelae include root dilaceration and ectopic eruption of the permanent successor [10].

5.2.5 Behavior Guidance

A clinical examination for this type of injury for any age child, including those with special health care needs can be done in the traditional dental setting. For very young children, a knee-to-knee exam with a caregiver provides good visibility of the oral cavity. Caregivers are asked to assist with hands and feet during the examination. For young children, an occlusal radiograph can be made with the child sitting on the caregiver's lap. The caregiver is instructed to hold the child's head and the film once it is positioned in the mouth.

If the treatment of choice is to allow spontaneous repositioning, no additional treatment is needed at the initial visit.

If the tooth or teeth are repositioned or extracted, a combination of non-pharmacologic and pharmacologic behavior guidance techniques can be used. Both the repositioning and the extraction are relatively quick procedures, so nitrous oxide inhalation or minimal sedation should be sufficient.

5.3 Extrusive Luxation

This type of dental trauma results in the tooth being extruded part of the way out of the socket. The clinical appearance is of the tooth being elongated (Fig. 5.5). It is also likely to be sensitive to percussion. Because it is partially or mostly out of the

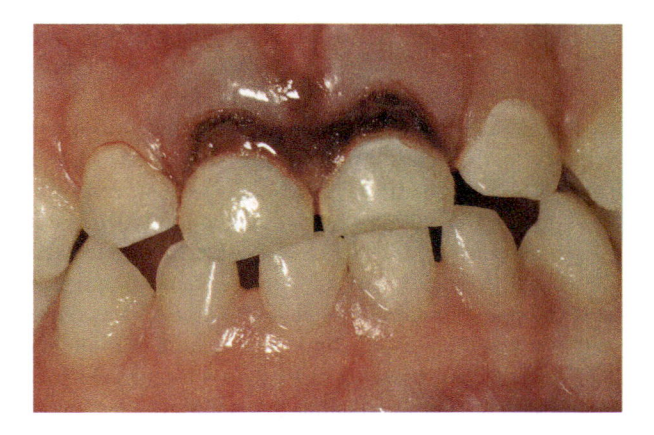

Fig. 5.5 Extrusion of primary central incisors. Repositioning teeth should be attempted

alveolar bone, it is also very mobile. Diagnosis is made by clinical and radiographic examination. The clinical exam should rule out any alveolar fracture and intraoral radiographs are made to rule out root fracture and to assess the degree of root development.

5.3.1 Treatment Recommendations

The treatment decision depends on the extent of extrusion, the level of root development, elapsed time since the injury and the behavior of the child. The IADT Guidelines recommend extraction for extrusion greater than 3 mm in teeth with fully formed, closed apex [2]. If the tooth is immature with an open apex and the extrusion is less than 3 mm, repositioning is recommended. Other factors to consider are whether the child uses a pacifier or has a finger or thumb sucking habit. In these cases, it is unlikely that the repositioned tooth will regain stability. If there has been a significant delay since the injury occurred, it may be difficult to reposition the tooth because of the coagulum in the socket. Extraction should be considered in these situations.

5.3.2 Follow-Up

It is important to monitor the vitality of the tooth, the continued root development and the eruption path of the permanent successor. A clinical exam should be completed at 1 week and a clinical and radiographic examination at 6–8 weeks, 6 months, and 1 year should be done [2].

5.3.3 Prognosis

The prognosis of the primary teeth is dependent on the severity of the injury. Repositioned primary teeth can return to physiologic mobility if given time without additional forces from chewing, biting, and non-nutritive sucking habits. There is a risk for discoloration and pulp necrosis with this type of injury, so regular monitoring is indicated.

In a study of healing complications related to lateral and extrusive luxations of primary teeth, Lauridsen et al. reported on the risk for pulp necrosis (PN), pulp canal obliteration (PCO), infection-related resorption (IRR), ankylosis-related resorption (ARR), repair-related resorption (RRR), and premature tooth loss (PTL) [7]. In many cases, extruded incisors were extracted at the time of injury. Among the 26 teeth with extrusive luxation that were not extracted, all were repositioned manually and not splinted. Pulp canal obliteration was diagnosed radiographically. Pulp necrosis was diagnosed with a combination of clinical and radiographic findings. If a primary incisor was lost more than 4 months earlier than the non-injured contralateral tooth, it was defined as premature tooth loss. The most common complication was premature tooth loss (43.3%), followed by pulp canal obliteration (39.8%) and pulp necrosis (15.6%). There were no cases of ankylosis-related resorption and the risk for repair-related resorption and infection-related resorption was 4.4% and 3.8%, respectively [7]. These findings support taking a conservative approach to the management of extrusive injuries of primary teeth and of maintaining a regular follow-up schedule so that any signs of pulp necrosis or infection-related resorption is detected and managed in a timely way.

In another study of luxated primary teeth, Soporowski et al. reported that extrusive luxations were the least common type of luxation in their study group [8]. In this sample, 50% of the teeth were observed, 11.5% were repositioned, and 38.5% were extracted. There were no enamel defects seen in permanent tooth successors following extrusive injuries [8].

Data reported in the IADT Trauma Guide is similar to that reported in other studies. After 3 years, the risk of tooth loss was 77%, the risk for pulp canal obliteration was >16% and for pulp necrosis was 6.4% [9].

5.3.4   Sequelae

Sequelae for the primary tooth include premature tooth loss, pulp necrosis, calcific metamorphosis, and inflammatory root resorption. For the permanent successor, there is a risk of enamel defects such as opacity or enamel hypoplasia, particularly if the primary tooth is repositioned resulting in the primary tooth root contacting the developing permanent tooth crown. The permanent tooth is also at risk for developmental defects if the primary tooth becomes abscessed and is not managed in a timely way.

5.3.5   Behavior Guidance

A clinical examination for this type of injury for any age child, including those with special health care needs can be done in the traditional dental setting. For very young children, a knee-to-knee exam with a caregiver provides good visibility of the oral cavity. Caregivers are asked to assist with hands and feet during the examination. For young children, an occlusal radiograph can be made with the child sitting on the caregiver's lap. The caregiver is instructed to hold the child's head and the film once it is positioned in the mouth.

If the treatment of choice is to allow spontaneous repositioning, no additional treatment is needed at the initial visit.

If the tooth or teeth are repositioned or extracted, a combination of non-pharmacologic and pharmacologic behavior guidance techniques can be used. Both the repositioning and the extraction are relatively quick procedures, so nitrous oxide inhalation or minimal sedation should be sufficient.

5.4   Intrusive Luxation

This dental injury occurs when the tooth is displaced into the socket and often results in the root apex being pushed through the buccal plate of the alveolar bone. This is a serious injury for both the primary tooth and the permanent successor due to the position of the developing permanent tooth bud. In cases of severe intrusion, it may appear clinically as if the tooth has been avulsed or fractured below the gum line (Fig. 5.6a). It is also common for the upper lip to appear swollen. A radiograph is essential to assess the severity of the injury. And to rule out avulsion if the incisal edge is not visible (Fig. 5.6b).

Diagnosis is made with a combination of the clinical and radiographic examination. An occlusal radiograph is usually sufficient, but it may be necessary to make a lateral extraoral radiograph as well. One study of the diagnostic value of lateral extraoral radiographs for the purpose of determining the position of the primary root

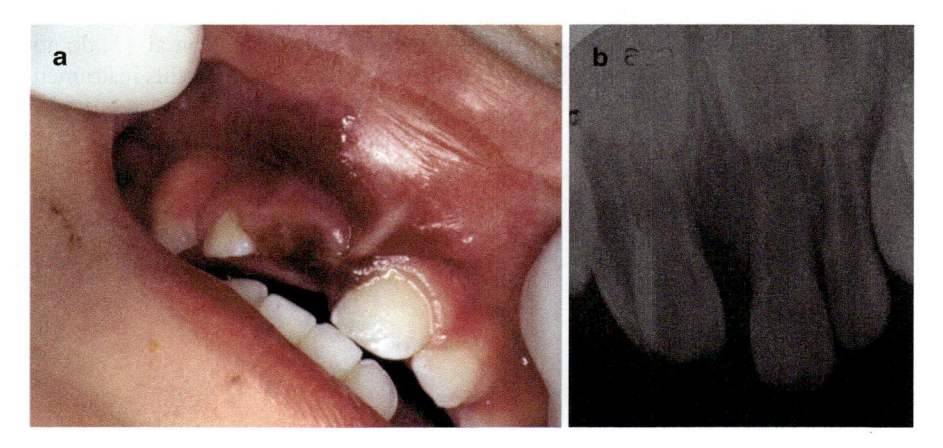

Fig. 5.6 Intrusive luxation of primary left maxillary central incisor. Clinically, it appears that the tooth was avulsed (**a**). The radiograph shows the tooth is intruded (**b**). In this view, it is difficult to tell the position of the root apex relative to the developing permanent incisor. External lateral radiograph was not attempted due to behavior

apex relative to the permanent successor found the value of this image to be limited [11]. Based on the radiographic findings, the clinician can determine if the root apex is positioned through the buccal plate, causing the tooth to appear shortened radiographically or toward the succedaneous tooth bud, causing the tooth to appear elongated radiographically.

5.4.1 Treatment Recommendations

The tooth should be allowed to re-erupt spontaneously if the apex is positioned toward or through the buccal plate. Measuring and recording the position of the intruded tooth relative to adjacent teeth will help to determine the extent of intrusion at the time of injury and if the tooth is re-erupting as anticipated. Re-eruption into the tooth's original position is expected to take 3 months [1]. This is variable and depends on the extent of intrusion, age of the child, and extent of injury to the alveolar bone. In the case shown in Figs. 5.6 and 5.7, the intruded incisor re-erupted spontaneously in 1 month. In a study of complications related to primary tooth trauma, Borum and Andreasen reported that 22% of intruded primary teeth failed to re-erupt after 1 year [12]. Four of the 15 teeth that remained displaced were ankylosed. A study of intruded primary incisors by Lauridsen et al., found that 83.7% of incisors re-erupted spontaneously after 1 year [13]. In the majority of cases, intruded primary incisors re-erupted spontaneously to their original position while the remainder were still intruded. When the primary tooth apex is visible through the gingiva covering the alveolar bone, the likelihood of re-eruption is decreased, and extraction should be considered. If the apex is positioned toward the developing tooth bud, it is recommended to extract the primary tooth to minimize damage to the successor.

Care should be taken when extracting intruded primary incisors to minimize the risk of damage to the developing permanent tooth or teeth. Flores et al. [1] do not recommend the use of elevators because of the potential for pushing this instrument

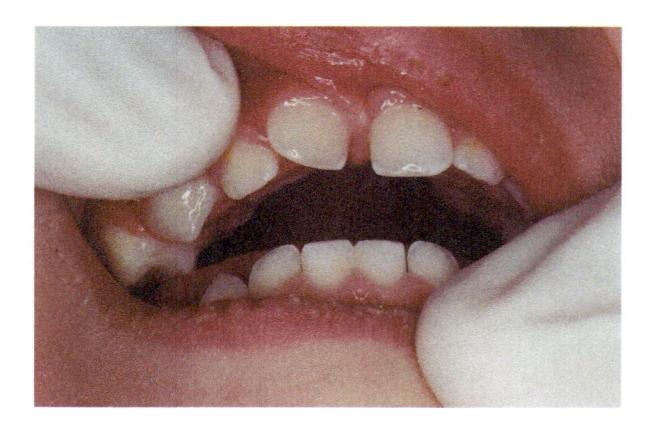

Fig. 5.7 One-month follow-up after allowing tooth in Fig. 5.6 to re-erupt spontaneously. Tooth was asymptomatic with normal mobility

into the follicular space. These authors also recommend using narrow forceps that allow the tooth to be held proximally and then putting pressure on the tooth so that the root apex is positioned labially to avoid contact with the permanent tooth germ [1]. Frequently, it is necessary to suture the extraction site to facilitate healing of the wound.

5.4.2 Follow-Up

It is very important for this type of injury to determine if re-eruption is occurring and to assess for continued root development and pulp vitality. The guidelines recommend a clinical examination at 1 week and at 6–8 weeks and clinical and radiographic exams at 3–4 weeks, 6 months, 1 year, and every year after that until the primary tooth exfoliates [2].

5.4.3 Prognosis

Prognosis for the primary tooth depends on the extent of the intrusion and whether or not re-eruption occurs. As in other traumatic injuries, discoloration may occur as well as pulp necrosis, ankylosis, or inflammatory root resorption. Lauridsen et al. summarized the findings related to 194 intruded primary incisors in 149 children [13]. These authors estimated the healing complications for intruded primary incisors after 3 years to be most frequent for premature tooth loss (39.4%), followed by pulp canal obliteration (38.9%), pulp necrosis (24.2%), and infection-related resorption (8.8%). The risk for pulp necrosis was the lowest for children under 2 years of age. The risk for repair-related resorption and ankylosis-related resorption were 3% and 3.6%, respectively [13]. These findings are in agreement with another study by Carvalho et al. who reported that pulp necrosis, premature tooth loss, and color change were the most common sequelae for both partially intruded and completely intruded primary incisors [14]. The most common age reported for intrusive injuries is between 1 and 4 years [14, 15].

During re-eruption, the child should be monitored closely for signs of infection in the area of the intruded incisors. If swelling and redness of the gingiva occurs or if pus is draining from the socket of the intruded tooth, the tooth or teeth should be extracted and antibiotics prescribed to minimize the damage to the developing permanent tooth [1]. The developing permanent tooth is at risk for enamel defects resulting from physical contact between the primary tooth root and the permanent tooth bud and from infection or inflammation that may occur as a result of the trauma. The prognosis is better for immature primary teeth than for fully developed teeth.

In some cases, an intruded primary tooth may become ankylosed. The IADT Trauma Guide reports a risk of ankylosis in primary intruded teeth of 3.6% [9]. Ankylosis of a primary incisor may result in a slight delay in exfoliation but should not require intervention.

5.4.4   Sequelae

The sequelae for intruded primary teeth are pulp necrosis, discoloration, and ankylosis. There is also a chance for an infection at the site of the intrusion, as discussed above.

For permanent teeth, enamel defects such as opacities or enamel hypoplasia are likely. In a study of primary tooth intrusion and effects on the permanent successor teeth reported enamel hypoplasia in 28.3%, crown or root disturbance in 16.7%, and ectopic eruption in 16.7% of the teeth evaluated [15]. In another study, de Amorim et al. followed 148 children with traumatic dental injuries to primary incisors until the permanent successors erupted [16]. As with other studies, maxillary central and lateral incisors accounted for the majority of primary tooth injuries. The greatest number of developmental sequelae to permanent teeth were related to primary tooth intrusions [16]. The number and severity of sequelae to permanent teeth was greater in children who experienced trauma at younger ages (between 1 and 3 years). Enamel hypoplasia and discoloration were the most common sequelae found [16].

Carvhalo et al. reported on sequelae for 66 successors of completely intruded primary teeth and 56 successors of partially intruded teeth [14]. Sequelae were present in 35.2% of the successors of completely intruded teeth and 53% of the successors of partially intruded teeth [14]. The most frequent sequelae for both were discoloration of enamel, disturbances of eruption, and crown dilaceration.

5.4.5   Behavior Guidance

A clinical examination for this type of injury for any age child, including those with special health care needs can be done in the traditional dental setting. For very young children, a knee-to-knee exam with a caregiver provides good visibility of the oral cavity. Caregivers are asked to assist with hands and feet during the examination. For young children, an occlusal radiograph can be made with the child sitting on the caregiver's lap. The caregiver is instructed to hold the child's head and the film once it is positioned in the mouth.

If the treatment of choice is to allow spontaneous re-eruption, no additional treatment is needed at the initial visit.

If the tooth or teeth are extracted, a combination of non-pharmacologic and pharmacologic behavior guidance techniques can be used. For a primary tooth that is completely intruded, a surgical extraction may be necessary to gain access to the crown of the tooth. Since this is a more common injury in the very young child, sedation of some type and possibly general anesthesia may be required to provide safe treatment.

5.5   Avulsion

Avulsion of a tooth is when the tooth is displaced completely out of the socket. Since a complete intrusion can appear as if the tooth was avulsed, it is necessary to confirm radiographically that the tooth is missing, not intruded. Also, if the tooth was not found at the scene of the injury, there is a possibility that the child swallowed or aspirated the tooth. This should be assessed through questioning the caregiver and observing the child for symptoms of choking or coughing. If aspiration is suspected, a chest X-ray is indicated. Both clinical and radiographic examinations are used to confirm avulsion of the tooth. The caregiver may present to the clinic with the avulsed tooth in hand or in a jar of milk.

5.5.1 Treatment

Replantation of an avulsed primary tooth is not recommended due to the likelihood of damaging the developing permanent tooth. Case studies have reported successful replantation and splinting of avulsed primary incisors and if attempted, this should be done with caution and with well-documented informed consent. A systematic review identified 19 case reports that documented 41 replanted primary teeth [17]. In 15 of these cases, there were no negative consequences to either primary teeth or permanent successors [17]. In 16 cases there were negative consequences limited to the replanted primary teeth, three cases had negative outcomes for only the permanent successor and in seven cases both the primary tooth and permanent successor had negative consequences [17].

In a critical review of this topic, Holan questioned the generally accepted belief that avulsed primary teeth should not be replanted and makes a case for the need for more evidence to support this and to provide guidelines for when replantation should be considered [18].

The IADT Guidelines recommend not replanting avulsed primary teeth [2]. Rationale for this includes the concern that replantation could cause damage to the permanent successor by pushing coagulum into the permanent tooth follicle or because of the likelihood of pulp necrosis and periapical inflammation causing defects in enamel mineralization of the developing tooth [1].

There is also concern regarding the risk for causing emotional trauma to the child that could result in post-traumatic stress disorder (PTSD) [1]. The injury is a traumatic event but replanting the tooth, splinting, and pulp therapy is also very traumatic for a young child. Studies in the medical literature have shown that unintentional injuries increase the risk of PTSD in young children. A report by Kramer and colleagues stated that 6 months after a traffic accident or burn injury, 13.9% and 10.4% of young children had PTSD, respectively [19].

5.5.2 Follow-Up

Follow-up should be done to monitor the development and eruption of the permanent successor. A clinical examination at 1 week and clinical and radiographic examinations at 6 months and 1 year and yearly until the permanent successor erupts are recommended [2].

5.5.3 Prognosis

In most cases, avulsed primary teeth are not replanted, so the prognosis for the primary teeth is clear. The concerns related to early loss of a primary incisor are primarily esthetic. It is not clear if the esthetic concern is more of an issue for the caregivers than it is for the child. There are limited studies that document the attitude of young children regarding prematurely missing teeth. Other potential concerns are related to maintenance of space in the anterior maxilla when an incisor is avulsed, and issues related to the child's speech. The few studies that have been conducted related to speech impairment and premature loss of primary incisors, suggest that if speech impairment does occur, it is usually transient and improves with the eruption of the permanent successors [20].

Evidence of space loss following premature loss of primary incisors is limited. Many reports are based on case studies and personal experience. One study of 167 prematurely lost primary incisors found that space loss occurred in only 2% of the cases [12]. Space loss in the anterior region is more likely if the incisors are lost prior to the eruption of the primary canines. In their review of this topic, Holan and Needleman suggest that space loss is greater: in the maxilla, if the dentition is crowded, if the tooth or teeth are lost early, the more posterior the tooth is in the arch (molars versus incisors) and the greater the number of teeth lost [20].

There is a risk of enamel defects on the permanent incisor, even if the primary tooth is not replanted. When primary teeth are lost prematurely, the eruption of the permanent successor is often delayed.

There are a few options for tooth replacement that can be considered, depending on the cooperation of the child. These are discussed later in this chapter.

5.5.4   Sequelae

For permanent teeth, possible sequelae related to primary tooth avulsion include delayed eruption and enamel defects such as opacities or enamel hypoplasia. In a study of long-term consequences of traumatic dental injuries of primary teeth on the developing permanent teeth, Tewari et al. reported that the greatest number of long-term sequelae were associated with primary tooth avulsion [21]. These defects included yellow or white discoloration of enamel, enamel hypoplasia, crown dilaceration, enamel hyperplasia, vestibular root angulation and lateral root angulation. Since the avulsed teeth were not replanted, it is assumed that these sequelae were the result of the impact on the maxilla that caused the tooth to be avulsed.

5.5.5   Tooth Replacement Options

Caregivers often feel strongly that their child will suffer physically and emotionally from premature loss of a front tooth. Options for tooth replacement are available and can be considered for patients who are cooperative enough to tolerate the procedures required to fabricate them. The two most common options are a fixed partial denture or a removable partial denture. The fixed appliance involves fitting orthodontic bands around the primary second molars, making upper and lower impressions and sending to the lab for fabrication of an appliance similar to a Nance space maintainer but with one or more acrylic teeth attached (Fig. 5.8). The removable appliance is designed like an orthodontic retainer with acrylic on the palate, clasps on the molars for retention and one or more teeth in the anterior (Fig. 5.9). These appliances are primarily for esthetics. Patients should be discouraged from biting into anything hard or chewy while wearing these and it is essential that they maintain good oral hygiene and come in for routine care so that the eruption of the permanent teeth can be monitored.

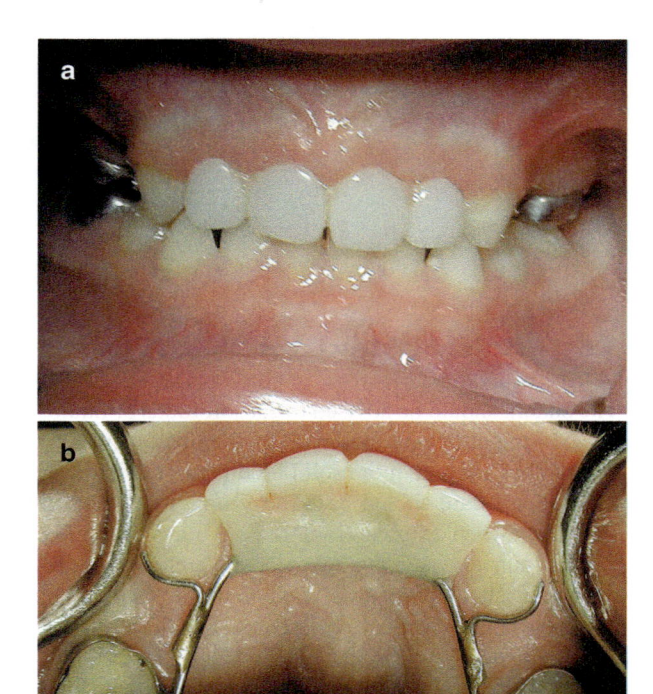

Fig. 5.8 Frontal (**a**) and palatal (**b**) view of a fixed partial denture that may be fabricated to replace missing maxillary central and lateral incisors. This requires cooperation for fitting bands, making an impression and cementing the appliance. It is also important that caregivers bring the child for routine check-ups so that the appliance can be removed before the permanent teeth begin to erupt

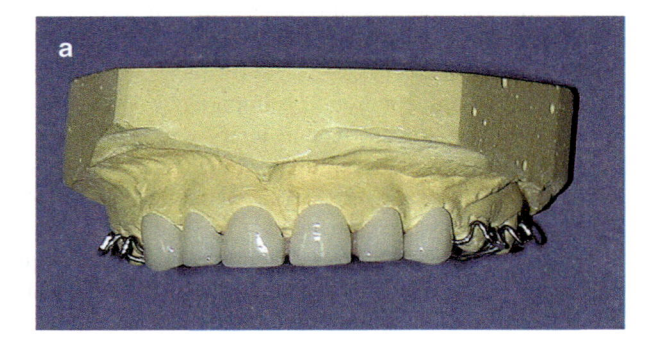

Fig. 5.9 Frontal (**a**) and palatal (**b**) view of a removable partial denture to replace anterior teeth. Clasps on the molars help with retention. This type of appliance requires cooperation for appliance fabrication and the ability to put the appliance in the mouth and take it out as needed

Fig. 5.9 (continued)

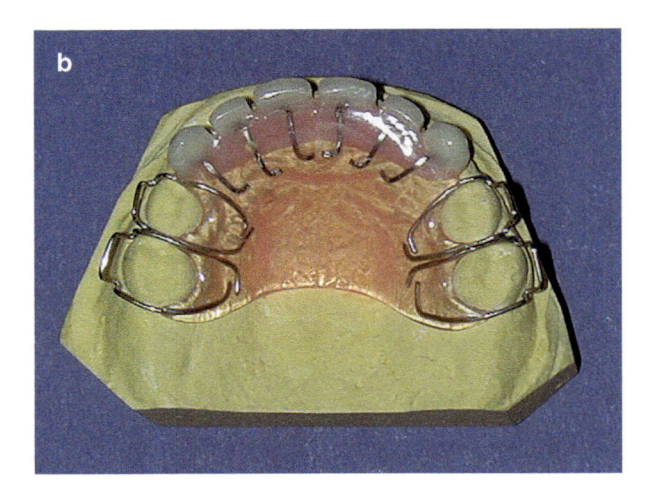

5.6 Patient Instructions

The patient should be advised to eat soft foods or liquids for 10–14 days. They should avoid biting or tearing food with their injured teeth for up to 6 weeks. After the first 2 weeks, they may eat more solid food if it is cut into small pieces. If the child is using a sippy cup, care should be taken so that they aren't putting undue pressure on the front teeth when drinking from the cup. It may be preferable to use a cup without a lid.

Non-nutritive sucking habits create a challenge for healing after trauma to anterior teeth. The habit is usually soothing for the child but increases the risk for additional trauma to the teeth or alveolus. Pacifier use should be restricted or eliminated during the healing process.

Good oral hygiene following a traumatic dental injury is essential for good healing. The teeth and oral tissues are likely to be sensitive, so a soft toothbrush should be used after each meal to remove food debris and plaque. The bristles can be further softened by running the brush under warm water before use. Alcohol free chlorhexidine (0.12%) should be applied to the teeth in the area of the trauma using a soft brush or cotton swab. Older children who are able to rinse and spit should swish with chlorhexidine 2–3 times per day. This will minimize the plaque buildup in the area of trauma [9].

For very young children, it is important to prevent a second injury while the first injury is still healing. A second injury will negatively impact the prognosis of the injured teeth. For older children who are involved in sports activities, it is best to avoid these activities for 2–3 weeks and then wear a protective mouthguard once the sporting activity has begun again.

Advice about possible complications and future sequelae should be provided to the caregiver. It may be beneficial to have this information in written form that the family can take home and refer to at a later time. It can also be available on the clinic's website. The signs to watch for during the first few weeks include swelling, increased mobility, infection, or drainage from a fistula. Evidence of increased redness or infection should be a sign to return to the office for evaluation. Bleeding should be under control by the time the child leaves the office but if bleeding continues or starts again after returning home, the family should contact the office. As healing progresses, the caregivers may notice a change in the color of injured teeth (gray or yellow), swelling, abscess formation, increased mobility of the tooth, and/ or detachment of the splint (if present).

Children may or may not complain of pain. If pain is keeping the child awake at night or interfering with their ability to eat or drink, they should be given the appropriate dose of liquid ibuprofen or acetaminophen to keep them comfortable.

It is important to inform caregivers about any possible complications that may affect the permanent teeth. This should also be explained as part of the written documentation given at the time of dismissal.

References

1. Flores MT, Holan G, Andreasen JO, Lauridsen E. Injuries to the primary dentition. In: Andreasen JO, Andreasen FM, Andersson L, editors. Textbook and color atlas of traumatic injuries to the teeth. 5th ed. Hoboken: Wiley-Blackwell; 2019. p. 556–88.
2. Malmgren B, Adreasen JO, Flores MT, Robertson A, DiAngelis AJ, Andersson L, Cavalleri G, Cohenca N, Day P, Hicks ML, Malmgren O, Moule AJ, Onetto J, Tsukiboshi M, International Association of Dental Traumatology. International Association of Dental Traumatology guidelines for the management of traumatic dental injuries: 3. Injuries in the primary dentition. Dent Traumatol. 2012;28:174–82.
3. Cardoso M, de Carvalho Rocha MJ. Association of crown discoloration and pulp status in traumatized primary teeth. Dental Traumatol. 2010;26:321–4.
4. Holan G. Development of clinical and radiographic signs associated with dark discolored primary incisors following traumatic injuries: a prospective controlled study. Dental Traumatol. 2004;20:276–87.
5. Mendoza-Mendoza A, Iglesias-Linares A, Yanez-Vico RM, Abalos-Labruzzi C. Prevalence and complications of trauma to the primary dentition in a subpopulation of Spanish children in southern Europe. Dent Traumatol. 2015;31:144–9.
6. Lauridsen E, Blanche P, Amaloo C, Andreasen JO. The risk of healing complications in primary teeth with concussion or subluxation injury-a retrospective cohort study. Dent Traumatol. 2017;33:337–44.
7. Lauridsen E, Blanche P, Yousaf N, Andreasen JO. The risk of healing complications in primary teeth with extrusive or lateral luxation-a retrospective cohort study. Dent Traumatol. 2017;33:307–16.
8. Soporowski NJ, Allred EN, Needleman HL. Luxation injuries of primary anterior teeth--prognosis and related correlates. Pediatr Dent. 1994;16:96–101.
9. Andreasen JO, editor. The dental trauma guide. San Diego: International Association of Dent Traumatology; 2012. https://dentaltraumaguide.org/. Accessed 1/5/19.
10. Holan G, McTigue DJ. Introduction to dental trauma: managing traumatic injuries in the primary dentition. In: Nowak AJ, Christensen JR, Mabry TR, Townsend JA, Wells MH, editors. Pediatric dentistry infancy through adolescence. Philadelphia: Elsevier; 2019. p. 227–43.
11. Holan G, Ram D, Fuks AB. The diagnostic value of lateral extraoral radiography for intruded maxillary primary incisors. Pediatr Dent. 2002;24:38–42.

12. Borum MK, Andreasen JO. Sequelae of trauma to primary maxillary incisors. I. Complications in the primary dentition. Endod Dent Traumatol. 1998;14:31–44.
13. Lauridsen E, Blanche P, Yousaf N, Andreasen JO. The risk of healing complications in primary teeth with intrusive luxation: a retrospective cohort study. Dent Traumatol. 2017;33:329–36.
14. Carvalho V, Jacomo DR, Campos V. Frequency of intrusive luxation in deciduous teeth and its effects. Dent Traumatol. 2010;26:304–7.
15. Altun C, Cehreli ZC, Guven G, Acikel C. Traumatic intrusion of primary teeth and its effects on the permanent successors: a clinical follow-up study. Oral Surg Oral Med Oral Pathol Oral Radiol Endod. 2009;107:493–8.
16. De Amorim CS, Americano GCA, Moliterno LFM, de Marsillac MWS, Andrade MRTC, Campos V. Frequency of crown and root dilaceration of permanent incisors after dental trauma to their predecessor teeth. Dent Traumatol. 2018;34:401–5.
17. Martins-Junior PA, Franco FA, de Barcelos RV, Marques LS, Ramos-Jorge ML. Replantation of avulsed primary teeth: a systematic review. Int J Paediatr Dent. 2014;24:77–83.
18. Holan G. Replantation of avulsed primary incisors: a critical review of a controversial treatment. Dental Traumatol. 2013;29:178–84.
19. Kramer DN, Hertli MB, Landolt MA. Evaluation of an early risk screener for PTSD in preschool children after accidental injury. Pediatrics. 2013;132(4):e945–51.
20. Holan G, Needleman HL. Premature loss of primary anterior teeth due to trauma--potential short- and long-term sequelae. Dent Traumatol. 2014;30:100–6.
21. Tewari N, Mathur VP, Singh N, Singh S, Pandey RK. Long-term effects of traumatic dental injuries of primary dentition on permanent successors: a retrospective study of 596 teeth. Dent Traumatol. 2018;34:129–34.

Permanent Tooth Crown and Root Fractures

6

Fractures of the crowns or roots of permanent teeth are common findings and in the preadolescent child are more likely to be caused by falls, sports, collisions, and traffic accidents. In older adolescents, violence may also contribute to fractures of teeth [1]. In permanent teeth, crown fractures are more common than luxations due to denser alveolar bone and lower crown/root ratio [2]. As in the primary dentition, the maxillary incisors are the most commonly injured teeth and this risk increases when there is excess overjet. In addition, there are both environmental and behavioral causes of traumatic dental injuries. A number of studies have documented that children from deprived areas in England and Scotland have higher prevalence of traumatic dental injuries (TDIs) than the overall prevalence in these countries [3, 4]. In contrast to this finding, Da Rosa et al. [5] found that children in Quebec from the highest income quartile had three times the number of teeth with TDI compared to children in the lowest income quartile. There is limited data on the association between income and/or social inequality and traumatic dental injuries in the United States and other countries.

6.1 Clinical and Radiographic Examination

The details of a clinical examination for a child or adolescent with a TDI are described in detail in Chap. 3. Since there are significant differences between the management of children and teeth in the mixed and permanent dentition compared to the primary dentition, the examination details will vary for children with permanent teeth. One of the primary differences is related to pulp sensibility testing. This is much more commonly performed with permanent teeth. It should be noted that erupting permanent teeth, teeth with open apices, and teeth that have been recently traumatized may not respond to sensibility testing and this does not necessarily imply pulp damage or necrosis [2]. In a study of 121 traumatized permanent anterior teeth, Bastos et al. found that the teeth that did not respond to sensibility tests at the initial visit after a traumatic injury were more likely to have suffered from a

© Springer Nature Switzerland AG 2020
R. L. Slayton, E. A. Palmer, *Traumatic Dental Injuries in Children*,
https://doi.org/10.1007/978-3-030-25793-4_6

luxation injury than a fracture [6]. They also found that a lack of response initially was not associated with pulpal necrosis at the final visit and that the subsequent pulp necrosis was more likely to occur in displaced teeth [6].

Sensibility testing can be done with a cold stimulus, with electric stimulation or with Laser Doppler flowmetry. Many pediatric dentistry offices perform cold testing by spraying Endo-Ice (1,1,1,2-tetrafluoroethane) (Coltene Whaledent, Cuyahoga Falls, OH) on a cotton swab and applying the swab immediately to the tooth surface. It is recommended to test one or more of the non-traumatized teeth first to demonstrate to the child what the cold sensation feels like. In a study comparing the reliability of pulp sensibility testing with Endo-Ice and electric pulp testing (EPT), Jespersen et al. reported that the two methods were equally reliable in adult patients [7]. Some authors have suggested the use of Laser Doppler flowmetry to measure blood flow as a measure of pulp vitality. This technique has the advantage of being painless and more reliable in teeth with open apices [2]. Ahn et al. compared EPT only to Ultrasound Doppler Flowmetry (UDF) plus EPT in a sample of 246 teeth with a history of trauma [8]. They found that UDF was more sensitive in the assessment of pulp vitality in traumatized permanent teeth. Currently, the cost of this equipment makes it unlikely to be used in most pediatric dentistry practices.

6.2   Uncomplicated Crown Fracture

The term, uncomplicated crown fracture, is used to describe tooth fractures that include enamel and/or dentin but without exposure of the pulp. When limited to enamel, the fracture is visible clinically and there is no evidence of a concomitant luxation injury. To rule out root fracture, a periapical radiograph is indicated. Physiologic mobility is expected. The tooth is not expected to have sensitivity to palpation or percussion [9]. As was described in Chap. 3, a thorough medical and dental history is indicated after any traumatic injury. Use of a trauma assessment form should always be a part of the clinical and radiographic assessment. A form developed by the American Academy of Pediatric Dentistry (AAPD) is available from their website at: www.aapd.org.

6.2.1   Enamel Fracture

A fracture of enamel is visible clinically and there should be no evidence of exposed dentin (Fig. 6.1). Pulp testing is more reliable in children and adolescents with permanent teeth and should be attempted to determine pulp sensibility following a TDI. It is expected that the pulp sensibility test will be positive after a mild traumatic injury resulting in enamel fracture. If the tooth does not respond positively, this indicates that there could be damage to the pulp and a risk for pulp necrosis in the future [9]. If there are rough edges that may cause discomfort to soft tissues, these should be smoothed and restored using composite resin. No treatment is an option if the esthetics or rough edges are not a concern.

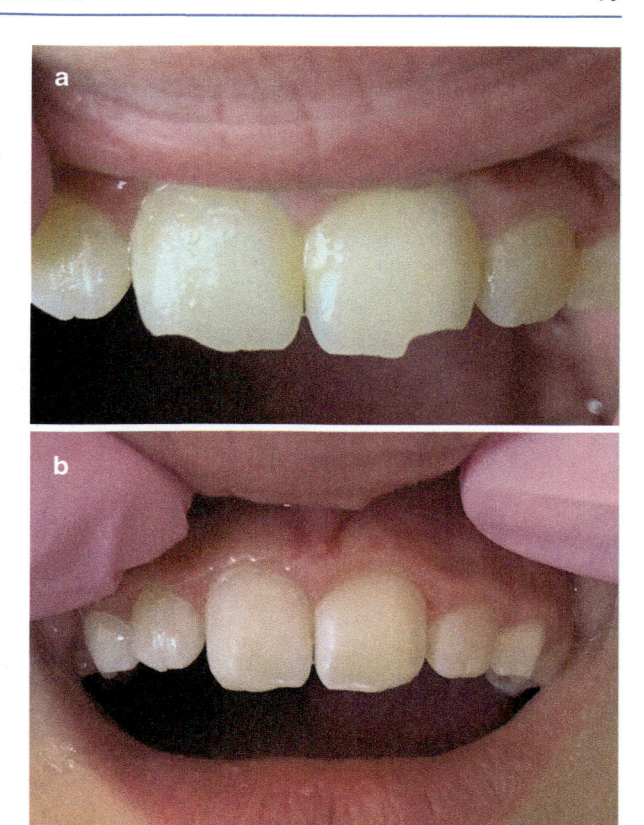

Fig. 6.1 Enamel fracture of permanent maxillary central incisors (**a**) restored using composite resin (**b**). (Courtesy of Dr. Purnima Hernandez and Bergen Pediatric Dentistry)

Unless there are concomitant injuries such as concussion or subluxation, the prognosis is very good. Olsburgh et al. estimated the prevalence of pulpal survival for enamel fracture in permanent teeth to be between 99 and 100% [10].

6.2.2 Enamel and Dentin Fracture

An uncomplicated fracture with exposed dentin is visible clinically and there is no evidence of pulp exposure (Fig. 6.2a, b). The tooth is not expected to be mobile but may be sensitive to stimulation such as changes in temperature and pressure and will most likely be sensitive to air blown on the tooth. Immature teeth and exposure of dentin closer to the pulp will result in increased sensitivity [10]. A periapical radiograph is indicated to rule out root fracture and establish a baseline. If the tooth fragment was not found and there is lip or cheek laceration (Fig. 6.3), a soft tissue radiograph may be indicated. Sensibility

Fig. 6.2 Uncomplicated fracture of the permanent left maxillary central incisor involving enamel and dentin but with no pulp exposure. Frontal view (**a**) and occlusal view (**b**). A temporary restoration may be placed to make the child more comfortable until the final restoration is placed. If the fractured tooth fragment is available, reattachment is a possibility

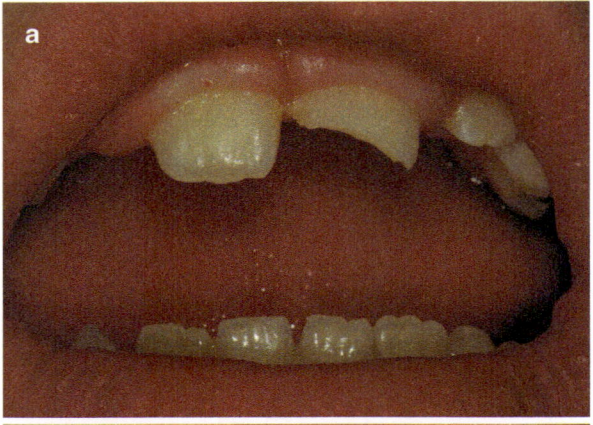

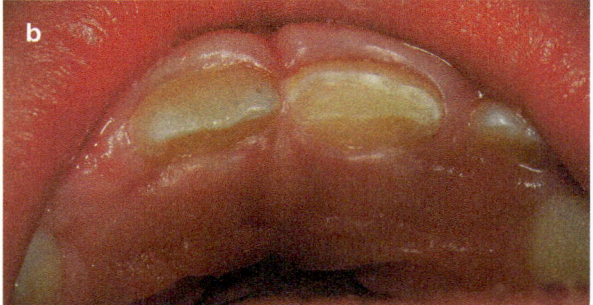

Fig. 6.3 Fractured maxillary incisors with laceration of lip. If tooth fragments were not recovered at the time of injury, a soft tissue radiograph is indicated to make sure the fragment is not imbedded in the lip

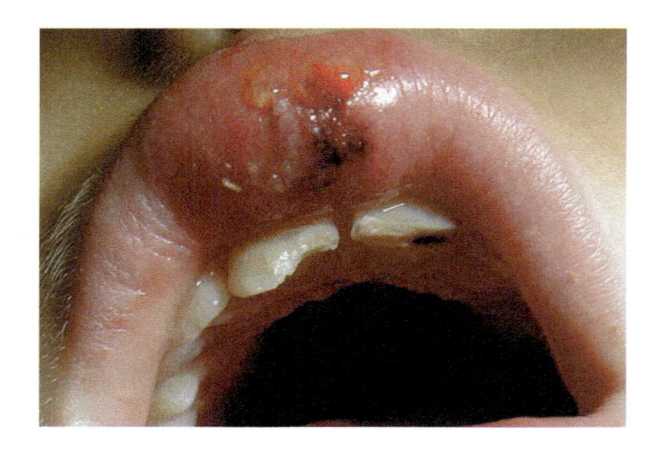

testing should be attempted but immediately after the injury, a negative response is a sign of transient damage and may indicate increased risk of necrosis at a later time. The pulp should be monitored over time at each follow-up appointment.

6.2.2.1 Treatment Recommendations

Inflammatory reactions in the pulp tissue are triggered by bacteria and their by-products. Exposure of dentin tubules provides a pathway for bacteria and other irritants to the pulp, putting it at risk for pulpal inflammation. The flow of dentinal fluid outward provides one mechanism to protect the pulp from bacterial invasion through hydrostatic pressure [10]. It is essential that all exposed dentin is sealed to prevent the invasion of bacteria. It is also essential to maintain the vascular supply to and within the tooth. Traditionally calcium hydroxide has been recommended but more recently, resin-modified glass ionomer has been used to create a strong seal prior to restoration with a composite resin. Some authors discourage the use of dentin adhesive systems on the exposed dentin due to the potential for pulp inflammation and delayed healing [2]. Other authors emphasize the importance of determining the remaining dentin thickness (RDT) prior to deciding whether to place a liner over the deepest part of the dentin or not [11, 12]. Trope et al. state that a composite restoration can be used as a restorative material with the traditional etching and bonding if RDT is more than 0.5 mm [12]. In a study by Costa et al. [11], RDT of 0.3 mm allowed diffusion of resin components into the dentin tubules resulting in pulpal inflammation. These authors recommended the use of a hard setting calcium hydroxide or resin-modified glass ionomer as a liner when there is a deep dentin lesion [11]. This is consistent with the International Association of Dental Traumatology (IADT) Trauma Guidelines [13]. When using calcium hydroxide, it is recommended to cover it with resin-modified glass ionomer to create a better seal and to facilitate bonding to the composite resin used for the final restoration.

If the fractured segment is available and is intact, it can be reattached following the protocol described below. If the tooth fragment is not available and there is time at the initial visit, the final restoration using composite resin can be completed (Fig. 6.4a, b). Often, the injury occurs after-hours and the dentist and family may choose to place a temporary restoration and then have the patient return at a later date for the final restoration. If this is timed properly, the first follow-up visit can be done at the same time as the placement of the final restoration. Delaying the final restoration may also increase the likelihood that the patient will return for follow-up due to esthetic concerns.

Reattachment of Crown Fragment

Reattachment of a tooth fragment after a TDI can be considered when the fragment is intact, can be adapted to the remaining tooth structure, and does not extend subgingivally. Hydration of the fragment is important, so it should be placed in a suitable medium at the time of injury or when the child arrives at the clinic. Recommended media for hydration include saline, Hank's Balanced Salt Solution, or milk. Every dental office and hospital should have one of these solutions on hand. The method for reattachment of the fragment is governed by the size of the fragment. Isolation with a lip retracting device and cotton rolls is recommended so that a dry field is maintained, and the dentist has good visibility, and access to the site of trauma. Using a lip retracting device instead of a rubber dam may also be more comfortable for the child, especially if local anesthetic is not needed for the reattachment procedure. For small

Fig. 6.4 Uncomplicated fracture of maxillary right central incisor (**a**) and restoration with composite resin (**b**). (Courtesy of Dr. Travis Nelson)

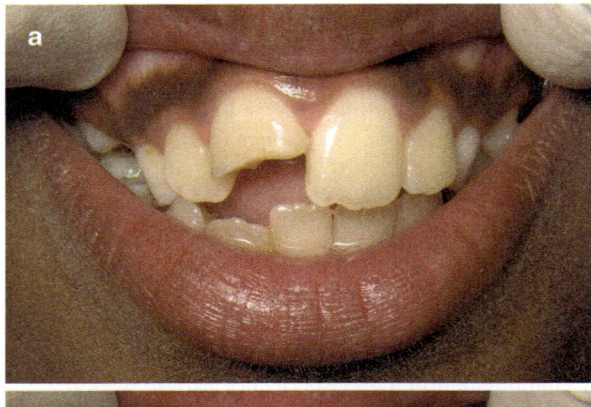

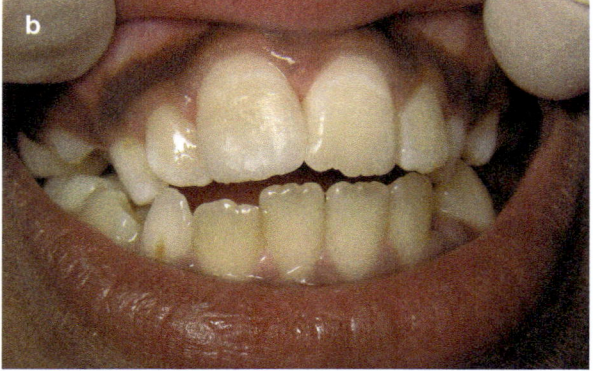

fragments, both the tooth and the fragment should be etched, rinsed and then an adhesive applied (Fig. 6.5a–e). Before curing, a highly filled flowable composite is applied to both the tooth and fragment (Fig. 6.5f). The fragment is then positioned on the tooth and light cured, finished, and polished (Fig. 6.5h–j) [14]. It is recommended to place a matrix between adjacent teeth to avoid bonding them together unintentionally. With a larger fragment, a resin composite should be used to attach the tooth and fragment together. In this case, the adhesive should be cured separately before placing the composite and positioning the fragment on the tooth. Once the fragment is repositioned, the composite is cured [14]. A third scenario can be considered when there is a complicated crown fracture and a direct pulp cap or partial pulpotomy is indicated. The modification of tooth fragment reattachment in this case will be described in the section on complicated crown fractures.

Advantages of reattaching a crown fragment are that the tooth is returned to its original appearance in a relatively quick procedure that can be completed at the same time as the initial visit for the traumatic injury. The disadvantage is that this technique has a relatively high rate of failure, necessitating a return to the dentist for reattachment or replacement with a composite resin restoration. In one long-term study, only 25% of re-bonded fragments remained in place after 7 years [15]. In a more recent study, Yilmaz et al. reported that 95% of reattached tooth fragments remained in place at the 2-year follow-up visit [16]. The tooth fragments that were

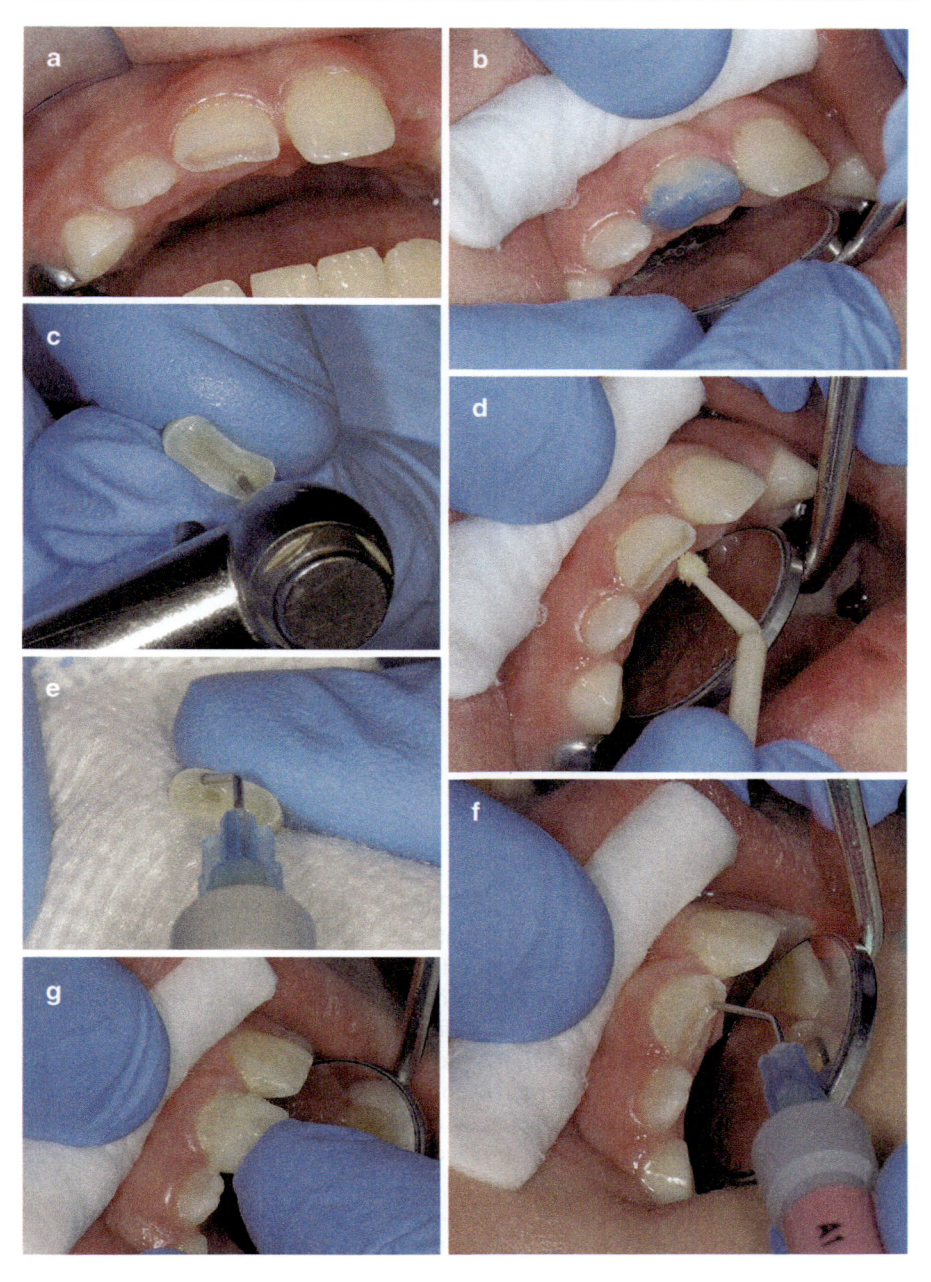

Fig. 6.5 Reattachment of tooth fragment in a central incisor with an uncomplicated fracture involving enamel and dentin. The maxillary right permanent central incisor has an uncomplicated fracture of enamel and dentin (**a**). Using cotton roll isolation, the tooth (and fragment) are etched (**b**), a groove is placed in the incisal fragment to accommodate the restorative material (**c**) and a bonding agent is applied (**d**). Flowable composite is applied to both the tooth and the incisal fragment (**e**, **f**). The fragment is positioned on the tooth and light cured (**g**, **h**). The tooth is then finished and polished (**i**, **j**). (Courtesy of Dr. Dennis J. McTigue)

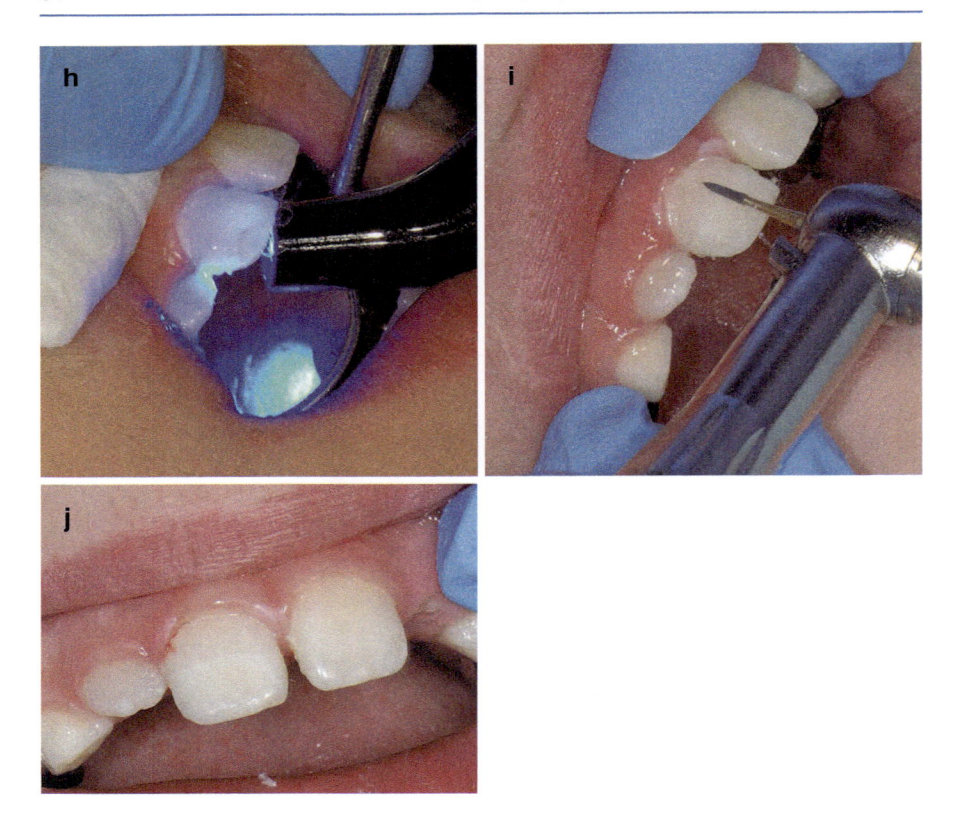

Fig. 6.5 (continued)

lost were due to a second traumatic injury. There have been a number of studies and case reports with varying methods and materials used for tooth fragment reattachment. In an effort to determine the most effective reattachment techniques for traumatized anterior teeth, Garcia et al. performed a systematic review of publications on this topic [17]. Of the 298 studies identified, 5 met the criteria for evaluation. The authors' conclusions were that tooth fragment reattachment following a dental traumatic injury is a reasonable alternative to composite resin buildups and that the preferred technique is simple reattachment using a composite resin rather than techniques that involve over contouring or placement of dentin grooves [17].

6.3   Complicated Crown Fracture

Fractures that involve enamel and dentin and exposure of the pulp are classified as complicated crown fractures. The injury is visible clinically (Figs. 6.6 and 6.7a, b). One or more radiographs are indicated to rule out root fracture and to determine the status of the apex (open or closed) (Fig. 6.8). A radiograph will also help determine

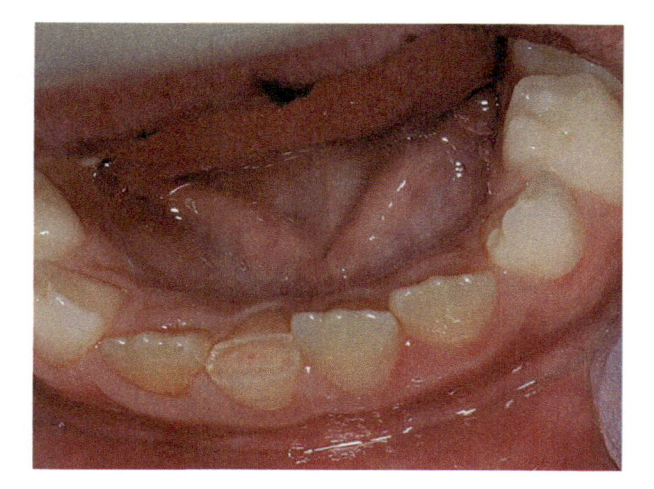

Fig. 6.6 Complicated fracture of the permanent mandibular right central incisor

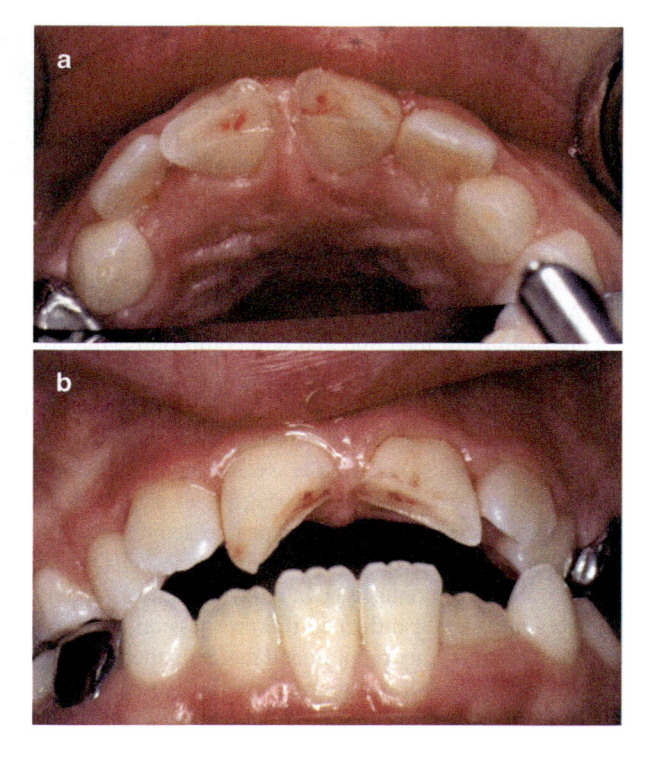

Fig. 6.7 Occlusal (**a**) and frontal (**b**) view of complicated fractures of both permanent maxillary central incisors

if there was a concomitant luxation injury. Treatment varies depending on the maturity of the tooth/teeth. If the tooth fragment was not found and there is lip or cheek laceration, a soft tissue radiograph is indicated. Mobility is expected to be normal and the tooth is likely to be sensitive to stimulation. Vitality or sensibility testing may not be reliable at the time of trauma but should be considered as one of the

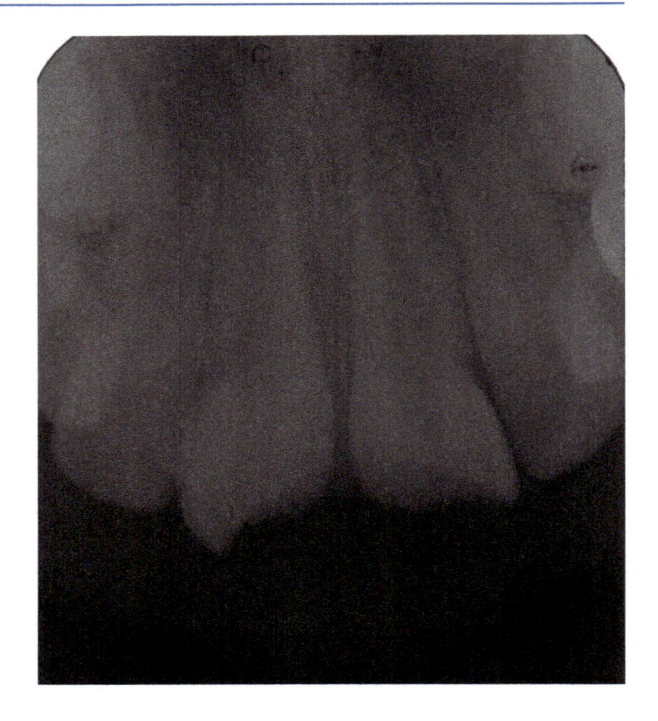

Fig. 6.8 Periapical radiograph of fractured permanent maxillary incisors. Apices are open and there is no evidence of concomitant injuries. Cvek pulpotomies are indicated

clinical evaluations. A negative response is a sign of transient damage and may indicate increased risk of necrosis at a later time [9].

A TDI involving a pulp exposure is viewed as needing urgent attention. It is most likely painful for the child and will compromise the ability to eat and drink. Because maintaining pulp vitality is one of the primary goals, covering the exposed dentin and pulp in a timely way is important. Studies of pulp exposures in monkeys show that the pulp is covered by a layer of fibrin in a very short time period. Inflammation spreads over time but does not usually extend beyond 2 mm in this model [18]. In a more recent study using a mouse model, He et al. found that pulpal inflammation began with a few hours of exposure and progressed rapidly [19]. At 72 h, necrosis had spread to the entire coronal pulp with inflammatory cells present in the radicular pulp [19]. It is not possible to do this type of study in humans, and it is unclear how the human oral microbiome would influence the progression of pulpal inflammation and necrosis. The IADT guidelines recommend that pulp therapy such as a direct pulp cap or partial pulpotomy be performed to minimize inflammation and maintain pulp vitality [13].

6.3.1   Treatment Recommendations

Treatment is dictated by the time since the injury, the extent of the injury, and the development of the root apex. Ideally, the child should present for evaluation within 24 h of the injury. For young patients regardless of the status of the root apex,

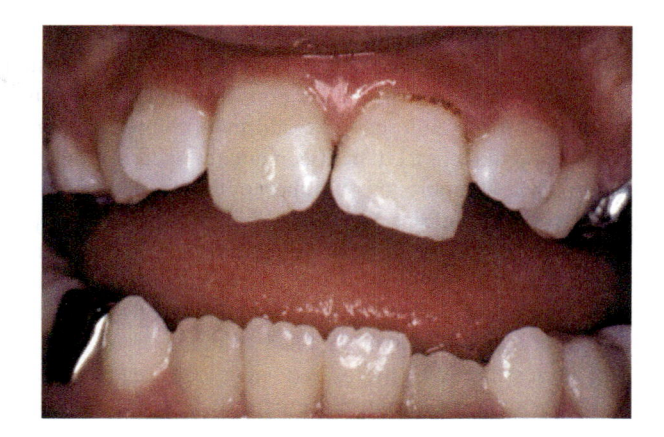

Fig. 6.9 Restoration of both central incisors using resin composite. This may be done at the time of the injury or at a follow-up visit after the Cvek pulpotomy and temporary restoration have been placed

maintaining pulp vitality is the primary objective. If there has been a delay in seeking treatment, it is important to establish the vitality of the tooth, if possible. It is also important to determine the restorability of the tooth. When there is minimal tooth structure present supragingivally, other options may need to be considered, including root canal treatment, orthodontic extrusion, and/or extraction. At the time of first presentation, if the trauma was recent and the tooth is restorable, the treatment of choice is a direct pulp cap using calcium hydroxide or mineral trioxide aggregate (MTA) for a small exposure or a partial (Cvek) pulpotomy for a larger exposure. If calcium hydroxide is used directly on the pulp exposure, it should be covered with resin-modified glass ionomer to provide a good seal prior to being restored with composite (Fig. 6.9). MTA does not require an extra layer, as it provides an adequate seal on its own. For anterior teeth, white MTA or a calcium silicate material should be used to minimize staining of the tooth. For closed apex teeth and older adolescents, if there has been a delay in seeking treatment, root canal treatment may be indicated [13].

In the last decade, a number of new tricalcium silicate materials have been introduced as possible alternatives to MTA. Some of these have the advantage of faster setting time and less risk of discoloration of the tooth. A comprehensive overview of MTA and other bioactive endodontic cements (BECs) for use in vital pulp therapy is provided by Parirok et al. [20]. They concluded that although some of the BECs show promise, the number and quality of studies comparing them to MTA are limited [20]. Kaur et al. conducted a literature review comparing MTA to Biodentine (one of the more recent BECs) and found that the advantages associated with Biodentine include faster setting time, easier handling, less discoloration and lower cost [21]. The authors also note that Biodentine is much less radiopaque than MTA, which is viewed as a disadvantage. Consistent with the findings of Parirok et al, the primary limitation is the lack of research to support the use of Biodentine in place of MTA [20]. As more studies become available, it is anticipated that this and other BECs will be viewed as viable alternatives for the management of traumatic dental injuries.

6.3.1.1 Direct Pulp Cap/Partial Pulpotomy

Complicated crown fractures in immature teeth require management of the exposed pulp to increase the chance for continued root development and pulp vitality. The success of direct pulp capping and pulpotomy treatment of traumatically exposed pulps in permanent teeth has been documented in a few studies and many more case reports. Many reports of pulp therapy focus on treatment of primary or permanent teeth with deep caries lesions. Although many of the principles are similar, pulp therapy in a vital, healthy tooth that has been exposed traumatically, presents a different situation than a tooth that has experienced chronic inflammatory insult from bacteria in a deep caries lesion. In the case of a complicated crown fracture, there are a few options for treatment and specific criteria for each option. All pulp therapy procedures should be performed using local anesthesia and rubber dam isolation.

Direct pulp cap is the placement of a medicament directly in contact with the exposed pulp without any removal of pulp tissue or dentin. Criteria for direct pulp cap treatment includes [10]:

- Duration since the traumatic exposure less than 24 h [22]
- Healthy pulp prior to trauma (no caries lesion)
- Diameter of pulp exposure less than 1.5 mm
- Open apex
- Absence of concomitant luxation injury

These factors improve the prognosis of this procedure. If there is a delay seeking treatment, the exposure is large, the tooth is mature or for some other reason, the pulp is not healthy, a partial or coronal pulpotomy should be considered.

Calcium hydroxide has a long history of use as a pulp capping agent because of its ability to form a dentinal bridge and its antibacterial action [10, 22]. It is placed directly over the exposed pulp and then should be covered with a glass ionomer cement prior to restoration. This will minimize microleakage. MTA is also a commonly used pulp capping material. In anterior teeth, there is a risk for discoloration, even with the use of white MTA. Other pulp capping materials include BECs, many of which have limited long-term clinical trials to support their use. After placement of the pulp capping material and ensuring a good seal over the exposed pulp and dentin, a permanent restoration is placed using composite resin. In some situations, it may be preferable to place a temporary restoration at the time of the injury and then replace it at the 1-week or 1-month follow-up appointment.

Pulp exposures that are larger than 1.5 mm or in cases where the treatment is delayed for more than 24 h, should be managed with a partial or cervical pulpotomy. A partial pulpotomy, sometimes referred to as a Cvek pulpotomy, involves removal of pulp tissue to a depth of about 2 mm below the exposure site, while a cervical pulpotomy involves the removal of pulp tissue within the crown of the tooth and possibly extending into the cervical portion of the root canal. A cervical pulpotomy should only be performed in mature teeth with irreversible pulpitis. In most complicated crown fractures, a partial pulpotomy will successfully remove the superficial inflamed pulp tissue adequately. The goal is to remove damaged tissue to the level of healthy pulp tissue. Healthy pulp tissue should appear red and bleeding should be able to be controlled by using a cotton pellet with pressure. If the pulp is hyperemic, that is a sign that additional pulp tissue needs to be removed. Pulpotomy procedures should be done using local anesthetic and rubber dam isolation. The basic steps of the procedure are outlined below. Removal of the pulp is done with a diamond bur in a high-speed handpiece with water spray to keep the site from overheating. Once the level of healthy pulp is reached, the area is rinsed with saline and then a medicament is placed directly on the exposed pulp. Historically, calcium hydroxide has been the most commonly used medicament for permanent tooth pulpotomies following complicated crown fractures [22]. When this medicament is used, it is covered with a glass ionomer cement to provide a tight seal. More recently, bioceramic materials such as MTA have been used for pulpotomies. MTA is a biocompatible material that stimulates dentin bridge formation and provides resistance to microleakage. Multiple studies have demonstrated very positive outcomes when using MTA and because it does not deteriorate over time, it does not need to be replaced at a later appointment [22].

Partial Pulpotomy Procedure (Fig. 6.10a–e)
- Administer local anesthetic
- Establish rubber dam isolation
- Rinse the tooth with saline
- Remove 2 mm of pulp tissue using a diamond bur on high-speed handpiece
- Provide copious water spray during procedure
- Check to ensure healthy pulp has been reached
- Place cotton pellet with sodium hypochlorite on pulp until bleeding stops
- Place calcium hydroxide or MTA over exposed pulp
- Place a layer of glass ionomer cement over the dentin and pulp medicament
- Restore with composite resin or reattach crown fragment

6.3.1.2 Reattachment of Crown Fragment

Reattachment of a tooth fragment after a complicated crown fracture is similar in some respects to that for an uncomplicated crown fracture. It can be considered when the fragment is intact, can be adapted to the remaining tooth structure and does not extend subgingivally. Hydration of the fragment is important, so it should be placed in a suitable medium at the time of injury or when the child arrives at the clinic. Recommended media for hydration include saline, Hank's Balanced Salt Solution, or milk. Every dental office and hospital should have one of these solutions on hand. The method for reattachment of the fragment is governed by the size of the fragment. Isolation with a rubber dam is strongly recommended since the pulp is exposed and the goal is to minimize contamination during the pulp treatment. As with the fragment attachment described previously, it is also important to maintain a dry field. Local anesthesia is indicated for the comfort of the child during this procedure. For complicated crown fractures, there is likely to be a large tooth fragment involved. The first procedure after anesthetizing and isolating the tooth or teeth is to perform a direct pulp cap or pulpotomy, depending on the size of the

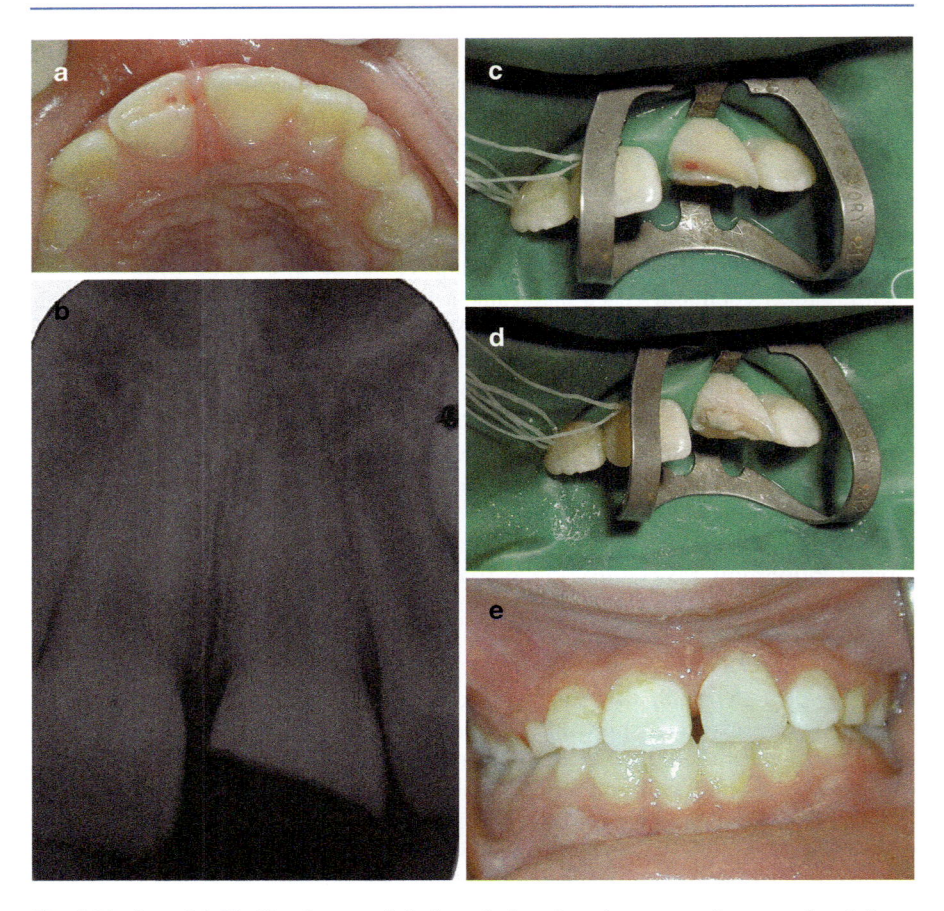

Fig. 6.10 A partial (Cvek) pulpotomy is indicated when the pulp exposure is greater than 1.5 mm or when the treatment is delayed more than 24 h. A pulp exposure is evident on the incisal of the maxillary left permanent incisor (**a**). The periapical radiograph shows there is no evidence of root fracture and that the apex is open (**b**). Rubber dam isolation is essential to minimize contamination (**c**). After removing 1–2 mm of pulp tissue, calcium hydroxide or MTA is placed over the exposed pulp (**d**). The tooth is restored with composite resin, ensuring that a good seal is present (**e**)

exposure. This procedure is described in a previous section. Once the pulp therapy is complete, the tooth and fragment are prepared for reattachment (Fig. 6.11a–g). It is usually necessary to modify the internal portion of the fragment to accommodate material that was placed over the pulp exposure. The fragment and tooth are etched, rinsed, and dried and then the bonding agent is placed on both surfaces and cured. Composite resin is placed between the tooth and fragment and the fragment is positioned on the tooth. The composite is cured briefly and then a chamfer is placed circumferentially around the tooth along the fracture line [14]. Then, additional composite is applied to fill in the chamfer to add strength and minimize the risk for staining along the fracture line. It should be made clear to the patient and the family

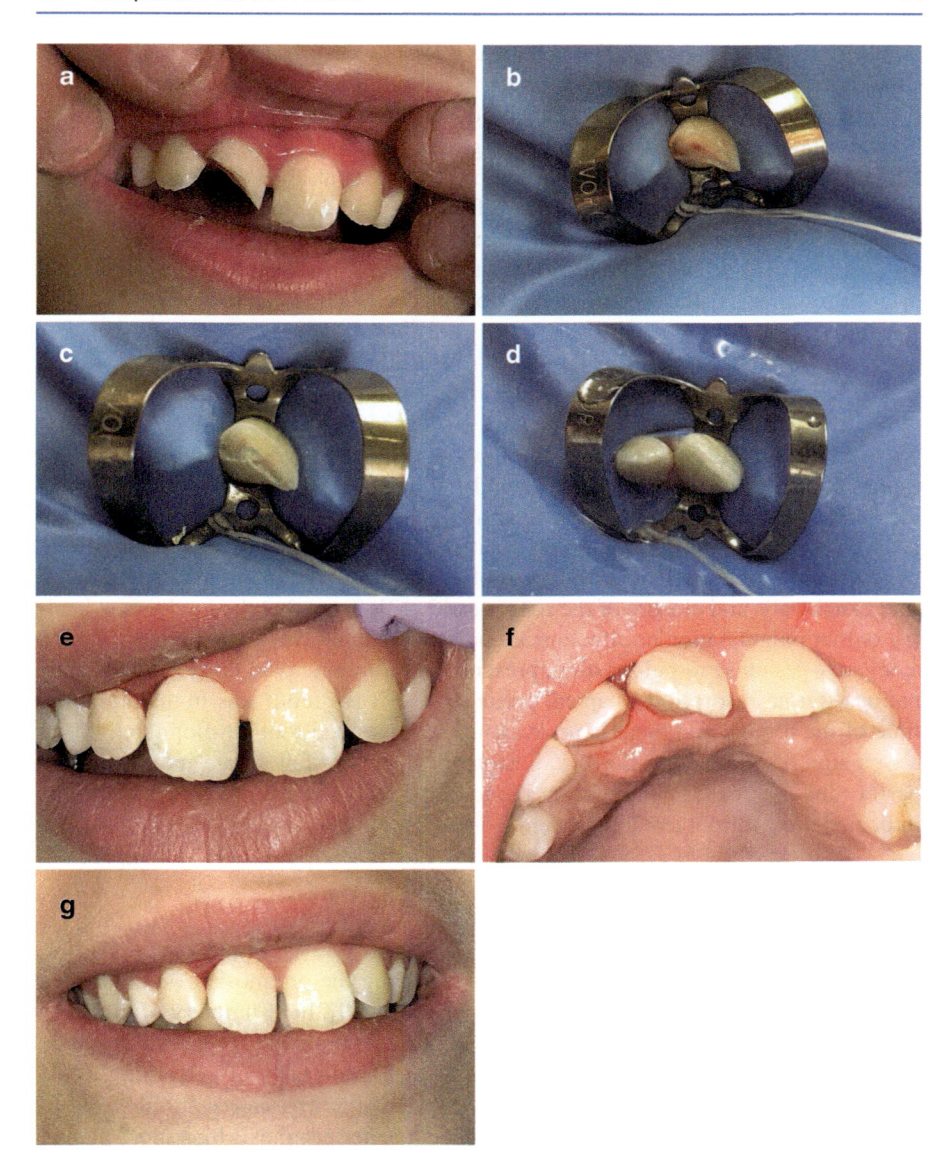

Fig. 6.11 Reattachment of tooth fragment for a central incisor with a complicated fracture. The pre-operative clinical image was taken by the patient's mother and sent to the after-hours attending dentist (**a**). After rubber dam isolation, a Cvek pulpotomy was performed (**b**). The pulp was sealed using NeoMTA (NuSmile) (**c**) and then the fragment was reattached as described previously (**d**). The restoration was finished and polished (**e–g**). (Courtesy of Dr. Matt Geneser)

that teeth that have been restored are not as strong as the original tooth and that care should be taken to avoid traumatic injury in the future. This is a good time to stress the importance of wearing a mouthguard during sporting activities.

Advantages of reattaching a crown fragment for complicated fractures are similar to those described above. In a study by, Yilmaz et al. of reattached tooth fragments in 22 teeth with uncomplicated fractures and 21 teeth with complicated factures, 95% of reattached tooth fragments remained in place at the 2-year follow-up visit [16]. The complicated crown fractured teeth were treated with a pulpotomy prior to fragment reattachment, as described above.

6.3.2   Follow-Up

The IADT Guidelines for fractures of permanent teeth recommend clinical and radiographic evaluation in 6–8 weeks and 1 year [13]. At these follow-up appointments, the findings that indicate healing and a favorable outcome are that the tooth is asymptomatic, and that it responds positively to pulp testing. For immature teeth, there should be evidence of continued root development including thickening of the root canal walls and closure of the root apex [2, 13]. Signs that the tooth is not healing or that inflammation or infection are present include being symptomatic, having a negative response to pulp testing, presence of radiologic pathology such as internal or external resorption or apical periodontitis. If the tooth was immature at the time of the trauma and there is no evidence of continued root development, this is also a sign of treatment failure [13]. Signs of treatment failure are indications for performing root canal treatment on the tooth. If the apex is open, apexification is indicated prior to root canal treatment.

6.3.3   Prognosis

There are limited long-term clinical trials regarding the prognosis of complicated crown fractures in permanent teeth with open apices [9]. In a summary of the prognosis of 16 teeth with complicated crown fractures, Andreasen [9] reported that only one tooth became necrotic after 5 years. Ravn [23] reported that in a study of 301 incisors with complicated crown fractures, pulp capping was successful in 90.5% of the cases. Teeth with immature root apices had a better prognosis than more mature teeth. Teeth with pulpotomy treatment using calcium hydroxide were 90% successful while 8.8% of those treated with zinc oxide eugenol resulted in pulp necrosis and 34.4% had other negative outcomes including pulp obliteration [23]. In a study of 375 teeth with complicated crown fracture, Wang et al. [24] reported that 10.1% of the teeth with partial pulpotomy and 9.8% of the teeth with coronal pulpotomy resulted in pulp necrosis during the study period (an average of 23 months). Teeth that received a direct pulp cap with Dycal were much more likely to become necrotic with a frequency of 57%. The frequency of pulp necrosis was higher with mature teeth than with immature teeth [24]. Pulpotomies were performed either with calcium hydroxide or MTA and no difference was found between the two materials relative to survival of the pulp.

In the classic study by Cvek [25] on partial pulpotomies and pulp capping for permanent teeth with complicated crown fractures, superficial removal of exposed pulp tissue was performed followed by placement of calcium hydroxide. There were 60 teeth in the study group and 96% of the teeth demonstrated healing after an average of 31 months follow-up. Healing was defined as the absence of clinical symptoms, no radiographic pathological changes, continued root formation of immature teeth, positive response to electrical stimulation and formation of a hard tissue barrier at the site of the injury [25]. The teeth in the study had mature and immature roots, pulp exposures ranging from 0.5 to 4 mm and the time delay before receiving treatment ranged from 1 to 2160 h. None of these variables appeared to influence the frequency of healing [25]. This and other subsequent studies support the conclusion that the preferred treatment for complicated fractures in young, healthy permanent teeth is a partial pulpotomy and a well-sealed restoration.

6.3.4 Sequelae

The most common sequela related to complicated crown fractures of permanent teeth is pulp necrosis. Wang et al. reported that pulp necrosis is more likely in teeth with mature apices than immature apices and that partial pulpotomy was more successful than pulp capping [24]. When treatment fails, the sequelae may result in the need for apexification, root canal treatment or in the worst-case scenario, extraction of the tooth. In adolescent patients, tooth replacement options are generally limited to removable partial appliances until the individual is done growing. Once growth is complete, treatment options include implants or a fixed bridge. If the tooth or teeth are lost at a young age, a bone graft may be necessary before an implant can be considered.

Pulp canal obliteration is a fairly common finding in traumatized primary teeth but less common and more problematic in permanent teeth. It is relatively rare in teeth with crown fractures unless there was a concomitant luxation injury [22]. Pulp canal obliteration in permanent teeth will be discussed in more detail in Chaps. 7 and 9.

6.4 Crown-Root Fracture: Uncomplicated

In this type of injury, there is a fracture of enamel, dentin, and cementum. The fractured fragment extends below the gingiva and there is no pulp exposure. The fractured fragment may be very mobile, and the tooth is usually sensitive to percussion. A radiograph may not identify the apical extension of the fractured fragment. A cone beam computed tomography (CBCT) may be required to fully diagnose the extent of the fracture. Andreasen et al. state that the most common causes of this type of injury are falls, bicycle accidents, foreign bodies striking the teeth, and automobile accidents [26]. The fractured tooth fragment is usually held in place by the periodontal ligament and may not be obvious to the patient or caregiver. Premolars and molars may suffer from this type of injury as the result of a blow to the chin causing fracture of one or more cusps [26].

Periapical and occlusal radiographs are considered the standard of care for diagnosing and monitoring traumatic dental injuries. It is recognized that the 2D nature of these images creates limitations in the diagnosis of some types of injuries. A recent review by Cohenca and Silberman provides current criteria for when 3D imaging techniques such as CBCT are indicated [27]. CBCT is advantageous for diagnosing traumatic dental injuries when compared to other imaging techniques such as computed tomography and Magnetic Resonance Imaging because of its lower radiation, high resolution, ability to adjust the field of view (FOV), and cost of the equipment [27]. Crown-root fractures are one type of dental injury that may benefit from the diagnostic ability of a CBCT. It is often difficult to evaluate the extent of the fracture using 2D images. Treatment decisions rely on accurate diagnoses and the prognosis of a traumatized tooth is dependent on both the diagnosis and the treatment. CBCT units are becoming more widely available in oral surgery, endodontic and orthodontic practices. Patients that require 3D imaging may be able to access this in one of these practices or in a hospital emergency department.

6.4.1 Treatment Recommendations

Crown-root fractures of permanent teeth are one of the most complicated injuries to manage. The number and size of the fragments and the apical extent of the fracture line dictate the treatment options available. The treatment choices appear to be controversial, as demonstrated by findings of de Castro et al. in a study of treatment plans for crown fractures by restorative dentistry specialists [28]. The age and level of cooperation adds an additional layer of complication in an adolescent with a crown-root fracture.

Because of the complexities in diagnosis and treatment of crown-root fractures, it is advisable to take steps to stabilize the tooth or teeth at the time of the injury so that the best options can be considered. Definitive treatment is dictated by the clinical and radiographic findings. Temporary stabilization of the fractured fragment may be possible by bonding the fragment to the larger coronal fragment using glass ionomer cement. If this is not possible due to the child's behavior or discomfort, the fragment can be removed and stored in saline until the reattachment procedure or other treatment decision is made. In this case, the exposed dentin should be covered with calcium hydroxide followed by a layer of glass ionomer cement. This will minimize the child's discomfort until an appropriate plan is made.

For any procedures involving crown-root fractures, the following must be considered: effect of the fracture on biologic width, stage of root development, stage of tooth eruption, pulpal status, and the degree of adaptation of the fragment to the remaining tooth [29]. In most other injuries involving fractures of teeth, the primary concern is the health of the pulp. For crown-root fractures, the periodontal health becomes an important consideration as well. Most of the options described below are best accomplished using a collaborative multidisciplinary approach.

Andreasen et al. provide a description of four different treatment options for permanent teeth with crown-root fracture including indications, advantages, and disadvantages [26]. The most conservative option involves bonding of the fragment to the larger coronal segment. This can be considered when the apical extent of the fracture is minimal. The procedure is described by Eichelsbacher et al. [29] and involves anesthetizing the tooth and surrounding soft tissues and laying a flap to expose the apical extent of the fracture on the root surface. Hemostasis should be achieved prior to bonding steps. The loose fragment and the intact coronal segment are etched, rinsed, and a bonding agent is applied and cured. A light cured flowable composite is used to attach the fragment to the tooth. The tooth is cured from multiple angles and any excess composite removed with a scalpel blade. The flap is then repositioned and sutured in place. It is important to check the occlusion and make adjustments to reduce any occlusal interference [26, 29]. Non-resorbable sutures are recommended, as the patient will need to return for follow-up and suture removal in 10 days. The patient should avoid brushing in the area of the surgery and should be instructed to rinse twice daily with 0.12% chlorhexidine rinse.

Eichelsbacher et al. treated 20 teeth with crown-root fractures using this conservative approach. After 2 years, all but two of the reattached fragments were still in place. The two teeth with dislodged fragments were the result of a second traumatic injury [29]. The authors measured periodontal health over the 2-year period and found no compromise as a result of the adhesive fragment bonding. They concluded that the use of adhesive techniques to reattach tooth fragments after a crown-root fracture is a feasible alternative in patients that are healthy periodontally [29]. Jardim et al. used a similar technique to reattach a fragment that extended subgingivally but in this case, resin-modified glass ionomer was used to attach the fragment rather than composite resin due to the close approximation to the pulp. In this case report, the pulp maintained vitality at the 1 year follow-up and there were no signs of periodontal pathology [30].

A second option involves removal of the fragment followed by placement of a supragingival restoration. This is more feasible esthetically when the exposed root surface is on the palatal surface. The unrestored root surface may be more susceptible to bacterial invasion and subsequent pulp inflammation, similar to the findings with crown fractures that expose dentin [26].

Exposure of the apical extent of the fracture using a gingivectomy procedure converts a subgingival fracture into a supragingival fracture that can be more effectively restored [26]. This is also more likely to have esthetically acceptable results if the fracture is on the palatal surface of the tooth. Once the apical extent of the fracture is exposed, the tooth can be restored with composite resin. In older patients, a permanent crown is indicated.

The third option involves the orthodontic extrusion of the tooth so that the subgingival extent of the fracture is exposed and can be restored. It is essential that root length be assessed in advance to make sure this is a viable option. For immature teeth, maintaining vitality is a high priority. There have been a number of clinical studies describing this technique and its value for the patient, although many of these reports involve endodontic treatment of the tooth prior to orthodontic extrusion [31–33]. In a case report by Fidel et al. [34], attempts to maintain the vitality and complete root formation of an immature central incisor following crown-root fracture was unsuccessful. The tooth had been treated with a pulpotomy and root fragment reattachment prior to orthodontic extrusion. Subsequently, root canal treatment was performed, and the tooth was successfully extruded and restored [34]. In a second case report, O'Toole et al. [35] treated a mature permanent canine that had sustained an uncomplicated crown-root fracture, using orthodontic extrusion and adhesive fragment reattachment. The clinical and radiographic findings after 3 years remained positive [35]. From the literature, it appears that in many situations, root canal therapy may facilitate orthodontic extrusion of teeth with crown-root fractures. However, for immature teeth or in cases where there is adequate tooth structure to complete orthodontic extrusion without root canal treatment, this conservative approach should be attempted.

Surgical extrusion can be done instead of orthodontic extrusion as a fourth option; however, this is likely to compromise the vitality of teeth with uncomplicated fractures. This method will be described in the section under complicated crown-root fractures.

In some situations when traumatic injuries occur in young children or children with special health care needs, the techniques described above are not possible. It is important that caregivers understand all the treatment options and the potential short and long-term consequences of these options before making a treatment decision. There are also financial considerations that may be difficult to determine but that can influence a caregiver's decision regarding treatment for their child.

The options described above require multiple visits to the dentist and in some cases, multiple specialists to complete treatment. When this is not an option for a family, another treatment consideration is decoronation and root submergence to preserve alveolar bone in anticipation of implant placement once the child has finished growing. Decoronation is discussed in more detail in Chap. 9. The technique involves laying a gingival flap, removing the coronal tooth structure to the level of the alveolar bone, extirpating the pulp tissue, and allowing blood from the root apex to fill the root canal. Then gingival tissue is sutured over the remaining root and allowed to heal. Clinical and radiographic follow-up is done to monitor the replacement root resorption that will occur over the next year or two. Replacement of the tooth can be done on a temporary basis using a removable appliance with an artificial tooth. Once the individual has finished growing, a fixed bridge or implant can be placed.

Extraction is the final option and is recommended for fractures where the prognosis is poor and/or it is anticipated that the child will not be compliant for the multiple appointments that are required for the other options. Vertical fractures or fractures that extend beyond the level where extrusion can be done successfully are indicated for extraction [9]. For more severe injuries, this may be the only option.

Replacement of permanent teeth that could not be restored will be discussed in a later chapter (Tooth replacement information in Chap. 8)

6.4.2 Follow-Up

The follow-up recommendations depend on what treatment is provided. In general, the patient should be seen for clinical and radiographic evaluation at 6–8 weeks and 1 year [13]. Again, the limited data on this type of injury makes it difficult to provide clear guidelines on the best follow-up protocol.

6.4.3 Prognosis

Outcomes for this type of injury are dependent on the severity of the injury, the treatment provided and the compliance with follow-up instructions. There are limited, long-term clinical trials in the literature regarding the prognosis of uncomplicated crown-root fractures in permanent teeth. Most are individual case reports with variable results [9, 26].

6.5 Crown/Root Fracture: Complicated

In this type of injury, there is a fracture of enamel, dentin, and cementum with the pulp exposed. The fractured fragment may be very mobile, and the tooth is usually sensitive to percussion. A radiograph may not identify the apical extension of the fractured fragment. A CBCT may be required to fully diagnose the extent of the fracture. The etiology is similar for uncomplicated crown-root fractures. Common causes of this type of injury are falls, bicycle accidents, foreign bodies striking the teeth, and automobile accidents [26]. The fractured tooth fragment is likely to be mobile and the tooth is sensitive to palpation.

Periapical and occlusal radiographs are considered the standard of care for diagnosing and monitoring traumatic dental injuries. It is recognized that the 2D nature of these images creates limitations in the diagnosis of some types of injuries. As mentioned above, crown-root fractures are one type of dental injury that may benefit from the diagnostic ability of a CBCT. Complicated crown-root fractures and their successful treatment may benefit from the diagnostic abilities of a CBCT.

6.5.1 Treatment Recommendations

Crown-root fractures of permanent teeth are one of the most complicated injuries to manage. When the pulp is exposed, this adds another layer of complication but also provides additional treatment options. As with uncomplicated crown-root fractures, the number and size of the fragments and the apical extent of the fracture line dictate the treatment options available. The age and level of cooperation adds an additional layer of complication in an adolescent with a complicated crown-root fracture. When compared to the uncomplicated crown-root fracture, the complicated fracture requires root canal treatment and in immature teeth, apexogenesis or some other procedure to maintain vitality until the root has completed development.

Because of the complexities in diagnosis and treatment of crown-root fractures, it is advisable to take steps to stabilize the tooth or teeth at the time of the injury so that the best options can be considered. Temporary stabilization of the fractured fragment may be possible by first placing calcium hydroxide over the pulp exposure and then bonding the fragment to the apical fragment using glass ionomer cement. If this is not possible due to the child's behavior or discomfort, the coronal fragment can be removed and stored in saline until the reattachment procedure or other treatment decision is made. In this case, the exposed pulp should be covered with calcium hydroxide followed by a layer of glass ionomer cement. This will minimize the child's discomfort until an appropriate plan is made.

For any procedures involving crown-root fractures, the following must be considered: effect of the fracture on biologic width, stage of root development, stage of tooth eruption, pulpal status, and the degree of adaptation of the fragment to the remaining tooth [29]. In most other injuries involving fractures of teeth, the primary concern is the health of the pulp. For crown-root fractures, the periodontal health becomes an important consideration as well. In crown-root fractures with a pulp exposure, root canal treatment is indicated when the tooth can be isolated effectively. Most of the options described below are best accomplished using a collaborative multidisciplinary approach.

Andreasen et al. [26] provide a description of different treatment options for permanent teeth with crown-root fracture including indications, advantages, and disadvantages. These are similar for uncomplicated and complicated fractures except that in the complicated fracture, either partial pulpotomy or root canal treatment is done early in the procedure. The most conservative option involves bonding of the coronal fragment to the apical segment. This can be considered when the apical extent of the fracture is minimal. The procedure is described by Eichelsbacher et al. [29] and involves anesthetizing the tooth and surrounding soft tissues and laying a flap to expose the apical extent of the fracture on the root surface. Hemostasis should be achieved prior to bonding steps. For mature teeth, root canal treatment is done prior to reattaching the fragment. If the tooth is immature, a partial pulpotomy is done with the placement of calcium hydroxide followed by glass ionomer cement to seal the exposed dentin. The loose fragment and the intact apical segment are etched, rinsed, and a bonding agent is applied and cured. A light cured flowable composite is used to attach the fragment to the tooth. The tooth is cured from multiple angles and any excess composite removed with a scalpel blade. The flap is then repositioned and sutured in place. It is important to check the occlusion and make adjustments to reduce any occlusal interference [26, 29]. Non-resorbable sutures are recommended, as the patient will need to return for follow-up and suture removal in 10 days. The patient should avoid brushing in the area of the surgery and should be instructed to rinse twice daily with 0.12% chlorhexidine rinse.

The study by Eichelsbacher [29] described above did not specifically identify which teeth had uncomplicated or complicated fractures. The authors did demonstrate that adhesive reattachment of fragments in crown-root fractured teeth was successful and did not compromise periodontal health. This is one of the few case series of this type of injury and treatment. Other cases have been published that show the successful reattachment of tooth fragments in teeth with complicated crown-root fractures and most involve the use of a fiber post in the pulp space to improve retention [36, 37].

A second option involves removal of the fragment followed by placement of a supragingival restoration. This is more feasible esthetically when the exposed root surface is on the palatal surface. The unrestored root surface may be more susceptible to bacterial invasion and subsequent pulp inflammation, similar to the findings with crown fractures that expose dentin [26].

Exposure of the apical extent of the fracture using a gingivectomy procedure converts a subgingival fracture into a supragingival fracture that can be more effectively restored. This is also more likely to have esthetically acceptable results if the fracture is on the palatal surface of the tooth. Once the apical extent of the fracture is exposed, the tooth can be restored with composite resin. In older patients, a permanent crown is indicated.

The third option involves the orthodontic extrusion of the tooth so that the subgingival extent of the fracture is exposed and can be restored. It is essential that root length be assessed in advance to make sure this is a viable option. For immature teeth, maintaining vitality is a high priority. There have been a number of clinical studies describing this technique and its value for the patient, although many of these reports involve endodontic treatment of the tooth prior to orthodontic extrusion [31–33]. From the literature, it appears that in many situations, root canal therapy may facilitate orthodontic extrusion of teeth with crown-root fractures. However, for immature teeth or in cases where there is adequate tooth structure to complete orthodontic extrusion without root canal treatment, this conservative approach should be attempted. With complicated fractures, root canal treatment is indicated for teeth with mature apices but a partial pulpotomy is recommended for immature teeth.

Surgical extrusion is an alternative to orthodontic extrusion; however, this is likely to compromise the vitality of teeth with uncomplicated fractures and therefore, is only recommended for teeth with complicated fractures and mature apices [26]. The goal of surgical extrusion is similar to that for orthodontic extrusion in terms of converting the fracture into a supragingival position. This procedure was originally described by Tegsjo et al. using the term "intra-alveolar transplantation" [38]. In a subsequent report, Tegsjo and colleagues provided outcomes of treatment for 56 teeth with complicated crown-root fractures, demonstrating the success for this procedure in both young and adult patients [39]. The patients were followed for 4 years. Eight of the 56 teeth needed to be extracted due to additional traumatic or prosthodontic complications. The method was further developed by Kahnberg who reported on a 10-year follow-up of 21 teeth with complicated crown-root fracture treated with this technique. All but one of the teeth were successfully treated with no evidence of pathology [40]. More recently, this procedure has become known as surgical extrusion. It is described in detail by Andreasen et al. [26]. Timing of each step of this procedure should be carefully considered. The surgical procedure needs to be done as atraumatically as possible and is more successful if delayed 2–3 weeks to allow inflammatory processes related to the injury to resolve. Warfvinge and Kahnberg suggest that better results are achieved by delaying endodontic therapy for 3–4 weeks after the surgical extrusion [41].

On the day of the injury, the exposed pulp can be extirpated or covered with calcium hydroxide and glass ionomer cement as a temporary restoration. The fractured coronal fragment can be removed or stabilized in place to the apical fragment until a treatment decision is made. Once it has been decided to perform a surgical extrusion procedure, the patient should be appointed for 2–3 weeks from the time of the injury. At this appointment, a surgical blade is used to release the periodontal ligament (PDL) all the way around the apical fragment. A narrow elevator is used to gently luxate the root. Forceps are used to extract the root to expose the apical extent of the fracture margin and to determine if there are other fractures present. The root is replanted and rotated if necessary, to place the fracture margin in an optimal position. This may be a 45° or greater rotation. The apical fragment is then stabilized in position, either with a splint (if there is enough tooth structure available) or with interproximal sutures. If the pulp was not extirpated previously, it can be done at this time and then the opening to the root canal is sealed with zinc-oxide eugenol. The root canal treatment should be completed 3–4 weeks after the surgical procedure. The final restoration can be completed 1–2 months after the root canal treatment. In adults, the final restoration is a post-retained crown [26]. For adolescent patients, a fiber post with composite crown serves as a functional and esthetic alternative until the patient reaches adulthood.

In some situations when traumatic injuries occur in young children or children with special health care needs, the techniques described above are not possible. It is important that caregivers understand all the treatment options and the potential short and long-term consequences of these options before making a treatment decision. There are also financial considerations that may be difficult to determine but that can influence a caregiver's decision regarding treatment for their child.

The options described above require multiple visits to the dentist and in some cases, multiple specialists to complete treatment. When this is not an option for a family, other treatment considerations include decoronation and root submergence to preserve alveolar bone in anticipation of implant placement once the child has finished growing or extraction [42] (Fig. 6.12a–d). Decoronation is discussed in more detail in Chap. 9. The technique involves laying a gingival flap, removing the coronal tooth structure to the level of the alveolar bone, extirpating the pulp tissue, and allowing blood from the root apex to fill the root canal. Then gingival tissue is sutured over the remaining root and allowed to heal. Clinical and radiographic follow-up is done to monitor the replacement root resorption that will occur over the next year or two. Replacement of the tooth can be done on a temporary basis using a fixed or removable appliance with an artificial tooth or teeth (Figs. 6.13 and 6.14a, b). Once the individual has finished growing, a fixed bridge or implant can be placed.

Extraction is the final option and is recommended for fractures where the prognosis is poor and/or it is anticipated that the child will not be compliant for the

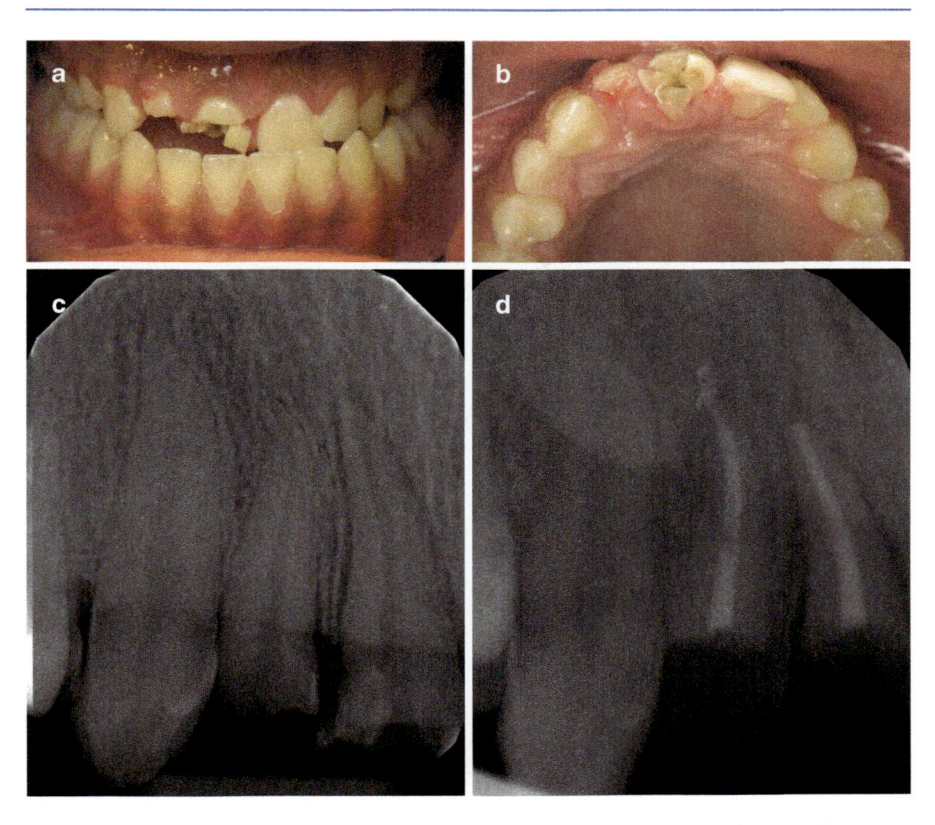

Fig. 6.12 Frontal (**a**) and occlusal (**b**) view of a complicated crown-root fracture. Treatment required removal of loose fragments (**c**), root canal treatment for the right lateral and central incisors (**d**), decoronation and root submergence. (Courtesy of Dr. Nestor Cohenca)

Fig. 6.13 Example of a removable partial denture to replace teeth #7 and #8. (Courtesy of Dr. Nestor Cohenca)

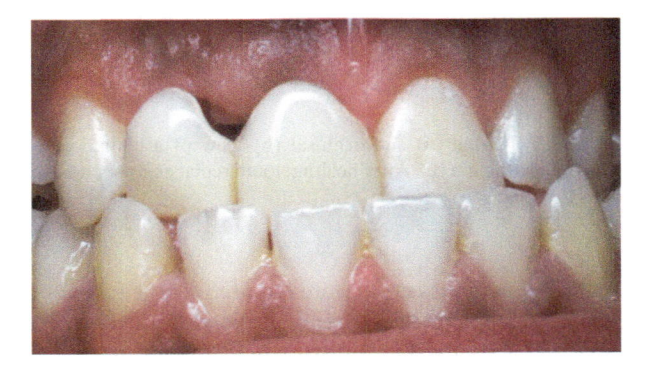

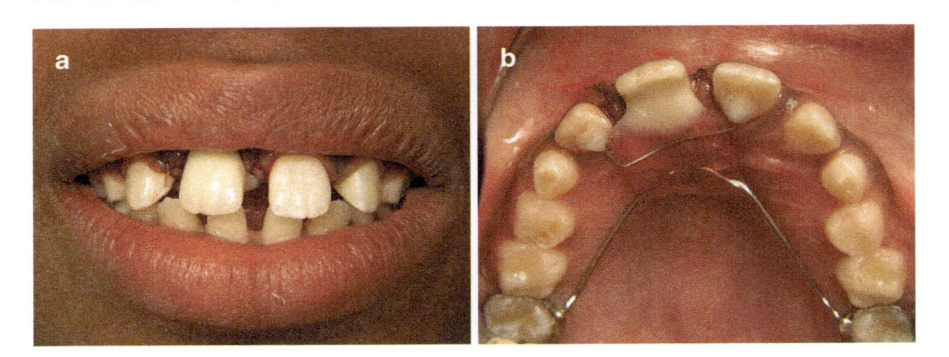

Fig. 6.14 Frontal (**a**) and occlusal (**b**) view of a fixed partial denture to replace tooth #8 after being extracted following trauma. (Courtesy of Dr. Travis Nelson)

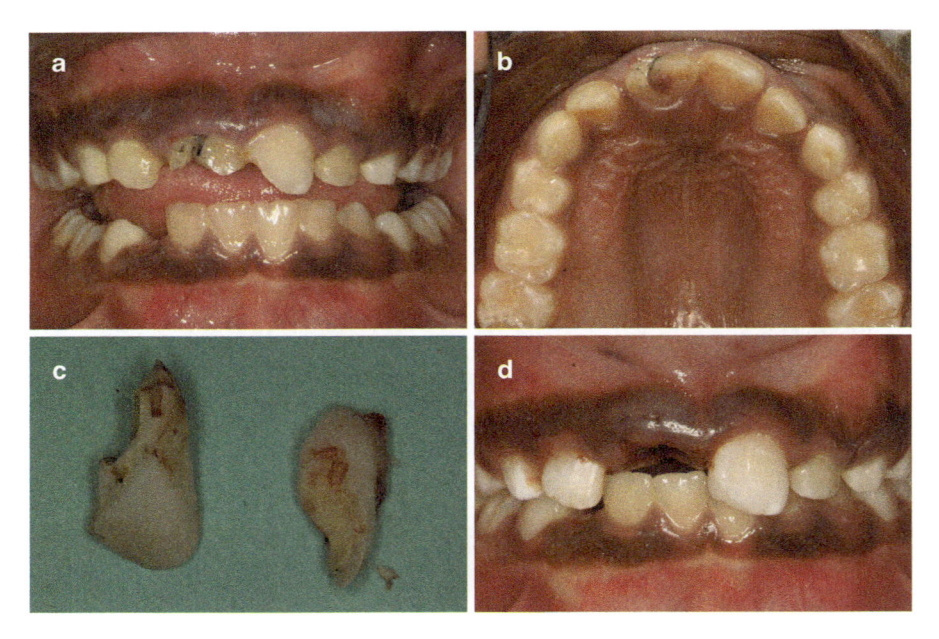

Fig. 6.15 Frontal (**a**) and occlusal (**b**) view of a complicated crown-root fracture. Treatment required extraction (**c**). After healing, tooth replacement options can be discussed (**d**). (Courtesy of Dr. Travis Nelson)

multiple appointments that are required for the other options (Fig. 6.15a–d). Vertical fractures or fractures that extend beyond the level where extrusion can be done successfully are indicated for extraction [9]. For more severe injuries, this may be the only option.

Replacement of permanent teeth that could not be restored will be discussed in Chap. 9.

6.5.2 Follow-Up

The follow-up recommendations depend on what treatment is provided. In general, the patient should be seen for clinical and radiographic evaluation at 6–8 weeks and 1 year [13].

6.5.3 Prognosis

The prognosis for complicated crown-root fractures is dependent on the severity of the injury, the treatment provided, and the compliance with follow-up instructions. There is limited evidence in the literature regarding the prognosis of complicated crown-root fractures with pulp exposures in permanent teeth. A systematic review of adverse events from surgical extrusion of complicated crown-root fractures found that the most common adverse event was non-progressive root resorption with a rate of 30% [43]. Less common findings included tooth loss (5%), slight mobility (4.6%), and marginal bone loss (3.7%) [43].

In another systematic review of surgical extrusion in permanent anterior teeth, Das and Muthu found that in cases of non-progressive root resorption, the incidence was higher when endodontic treatment was initiated before the extrusion procedure [44]. It is thought that this may be due to difficulties preventing contamination of the root canal during the procedure. There were no reports of ankylosis in any of the cases reviewed and normal form and function of the periodontium was seen in all cases. These authors concluded that surgical extrusion of complicated crown-root fracture in anterior teeth can be used successfully and has the advantages of needing less chair time, good esthetics, and a low incidence of failure.

6.6   Root Fracture

In this injury, the fracture is confined to the root and involves dentin, cementum, and pulp. It may also appear to be luxated. There is often mobility that is greater than physiologic mobility. One or more radiographs are required to evaluate the location of the fracture and the approximation of the two segments (Fig. 6.16a, b). In order to visualize a root fracture, the central beam of the X-ray head needs to be aimed in the range of 15–20° of the fracture plane [45]. Since fractures vary in location and angulation, it is recommended that multiple exposures with different angulations are made to maximize the likelihood of detecting a fracture [46]. There is no evidence at the current time to suggest that CBCT would significantly change the treatment plan for permanent teeth with root fractures [45].

Other clinical signs may include discoloration of the coronal segment and/or bleeding around the sulcus. The tooth is likely to be sensitive to stimulation, especially movement. The fracture is described by its location as in the apical third, middle third, or coronal third of the root.

Root fractures of the permanent dentition are relatively uncommon (0.5–7% of permanent tooth injuries) and are often caused by fights or the impact from an object [45]. The most frequently affected teeth are maxillary central incisors in children and adolescents between the ages of 11 and 20 years [45].

6.6.1 Treatment Recommendations

Root fractures are injuries of both the pulp and the periodontal ligament. The severity can range from being relatively mild with the two segments well approximated in the middle or apical third of the root (Fig. 6.16) to more extreme, where there is a significant gap between the segments (Fig. 6.17) or the fracture is in the cervical third of the root. In the ideal scenario, healing of the pulp and the periodontal ligament will occur over time. The best chance for pulpal healing is when there is no displacement of the fractured segment. This allows the odontoblast progenitor cells to form a dentin bridge connecting the two fragments [45]. Once this bridge stabilizes the fragments, cementum forms along the fracture line. Although this healing may be visible after 3 months, it is predicted to take a few years for the injury to be completely healed [47]. Hard tissue repair consists of dentin on the innermost layer and then an incomplete layer of cementum interspersed with connective tissue [45]. It is not uncommon to see partial pulp canal obliteration in the apical fragment [45].

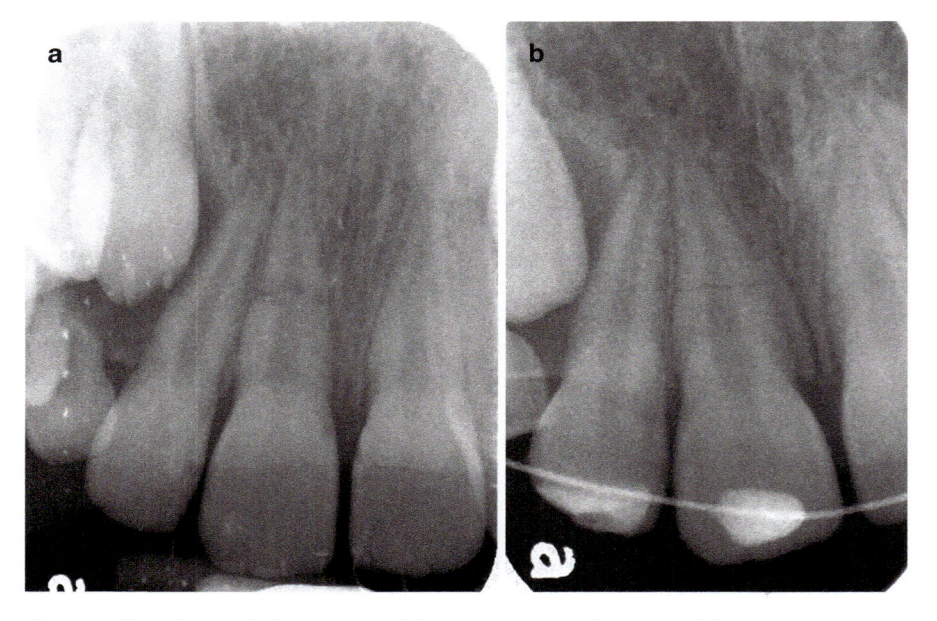

Fig. 6.16 Root fracture in the maxillary right central incisor. The location is in the apical third (**a**). After repositioning, a flexible splint is placed for 4 weeks (**b**)

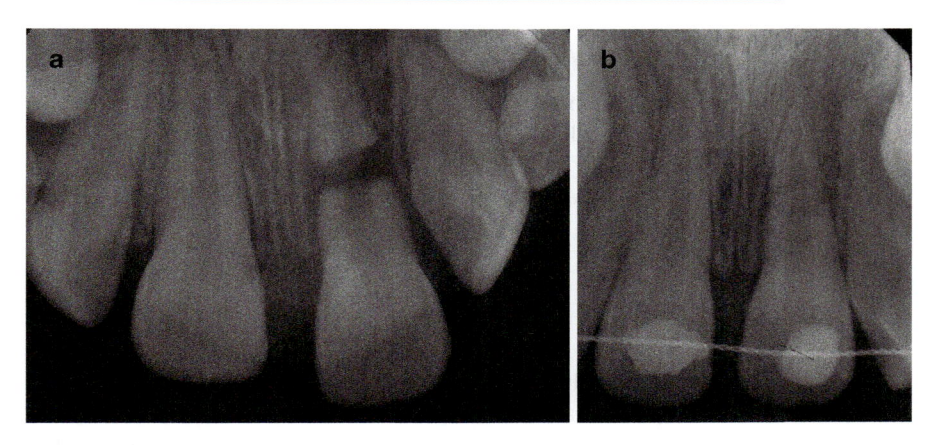

Fig. 6.17 Root fracture in the middle third of the maxillary left central incisor with significant separation between the segments (**a**). The coronal segment is repositioned and splinted in place for 4 weeks (**b**)

In a second scenario, when there is displacement of the fractured root segment, the pulp is either severed or stretched. Revascularization occurs in the coronal segment and periodontally derived cells grow into the space between the two fragments to create a zone of connective tissue healing [45]. The fractured surfaces in this type of healing are covered by cementum. Radiographically, this healing pattern appears to have a rounding of the fracture edges and a radiolucent line separating the fragments. The clinical findings will show slight mobility and a weak pain response to percussion. It is expected that teeth with this type of healing will have a normal response to sensibility testing [45].

Non-healing of the fracture site will result if bacteria gains access to this area. This leads to inflamed granulation tissue between the two fragments. If this occurs, the coronal segment will become more mobile and the pulp tissue in this segment is necrotic.

The coronal segment should be repositioned and stabilized as soon as possible in order to achieve the best results [2]. Verification of the position is done radiographically. The goal is to position the two fragments so that they are in close approximation to each other. Once in the optimal position, the tooth is stabilized with a semirigid splint for 3–4 weeks [13] (Fig. 6.14). The splint should be applied passively to avoid additional trauma. If the fracture is in the coronal third, a longer time period may be required. Pulp vitality should be monitored at follow-up appointments. When there are clinical and radiographic signs of necrosis or root resorption, root canal treatment should be initiated. Most of the time, the apical fragment will retain its vitality, so it is only necessary to perform root canal treatment on the coronal segment [2].

In cases where the coronal segment can't be saved and extraction is done, the apical fragment should be left in place. Over time, it is expected that replacement resorption will take place.

6.6.2 Follow-Up

For fractures in the apical and middle third, remove the splint in 4 weeks and evaluate clinically and radiographically. For fractures in coronal third, remove splint in 4 months and assess mobility and vitality. For all root fractures, continue follow-up at 6–8 weeks, 6 months, and annually for 5 years. Endodontic therapy should be initiated if the pulp is necrotic after 3 months [13].

6.6.3 Prognosis

Prognosis of root fractured teeth depends on degree of root development, degree of separation between fragments and on the position of the root fracture along the length of the root. Recovery from a root fracture involves healing of both the pulp and the periodontal ligament. Andreasen et al. reported on the survival rates of 492 root fractures and discussed factors that contributed to their successful healing [48]. The most significant effect on survival was the location of the fracture. The 10-year survival rate for root fractures in the apical third was 89% and for mid-root was 78%. Fractures in the cervical mid-root and cervical were 67% and 33%, respectively [48]. Type of healing also had a significant influence on survival. No teeth with hard tissue fracture healing were lost. In teeth with connective tissue healing, the 8-year survival for teeth with apical, mid-root, or cervical-mid-root fractures was greater than 80% but for cervical fractures was 25% [48]. When non-healing with granulation tissue was seen, survival for the apical and mid-root fractures was significantly greater than for the cervical-mid-root and cervical fractures.

Pulp necrosis and pulp canal obliteration are the most common findings for all types of root fractures [9].

6.7 Alveolar Fracture

Terminology to describe injuries to supporting bone include comminution or crushing of the alveolar socket, fracture of the socket wall, fracture of the alveolar process, and fracture of the jaw. This section will focus on fractures of the alveolar process.

In children and adolescents with permanent dentition, the most common causes of alveolar fractures are automobile accidents and violence [49]. In an analysis of 299 cases of alveolar fractures in the permanent dentition, involving 815 teeth, Andreasen and Lauridsen found that 44% of the injuries in men were from violence [50]. In women, 33% of the injuries were from violence, 32% from falls, and 26% from traffic injuries [50]. The maxilla was involved the majority of the time (74%) and the most common age range for this injury was between 15 and 25 years (43%) [50].

Diagnosis of an alveolar fracture is fairly straightforward because there is both displacement and mobility of an entire segment of the alveolus with multiple teeth involved. When testing the mobility of one tooth, it is noticed that adjacent teeth move as well. Often, the fractured alveolar segment results in occlusal interference. Many times, a fracture line is visible on the gingiva. Intraoral radiographs do not usually show the fracture line but should be made to identify other concomitant injuries. In some cases, a panoramic radiograph is indicated to rule out other injuries or jaw fractures.

It is expected that an injury significant enough to cause an alveolar fracture will also result in damage to the pulp, periodontium, and gingiva [49]. It is also likely that there are injuries to other parts of the body that will need to be evaluated in an emergency room setting.

6.7.1 Treatment Recommendations

Fractures of the alveolar process require repositioning and immobilization by splinting. Local anesthetic is required and for young or anxious patients, sedation may be necessary as well. Repositioning with digital pressure is usually adequate to get the segment back into place but if there is resistance, it may require slight extrusive pressure to unlock the root tips from the alveolar plate first. A flexible splint is placed using resin composite, an arch wire or nylon line. Bonding to teeth outside of the fractured segment is necessary for good anchorage. In the mixed dentition, this may require extending the splint to the permanent molars. The splint should be left in place for 3–4 weeks.

If there are soft tissue lacerations that require suturing, these should be done after positioning and splinting the teeth.

Alveolar fractures present significant treatment challenges for young patients and patients with developmental disabilities or cognitive challenges. In these cases, reduction of the fracture and immobilization with a splint may need to be done under general anesthesia.

6.7.2 Follow-Up

The splint should be removed in 4 weeks and at that time, both a clinical and radiographic examination should be done. Subsequent follow-up includes clinical and radiographic examination at 6–8 weeks, 4 months, 6 months, 1 year, and yearly for 5 years. Endodontic treatment should be initiated when signs of pulp necrosis are evident [13].

6.7.3 Prognosis

Factors that affect the prognosis of this type of injury are the maturity of the roots and the location of the alveolar fracture line relative to the apices of the roots. The most common outcome for permanent teeth with alveolar fracture is pulp necrosis and the second most common is pulp canal obliteration [9].

Lauridsen et al. evaluated the healing complications of 223 permanent teeth from 91 patients with alveolar fracture [51]. Five of the patients had immature teeth and, in these teeth, there were no severe complications. For the mature teeth, the estimate for pulp necrosis at the 10-year follow-up was 56%. Factors that increased the risk of pulp necrosis in these teeth was horizontal displacement of the alveolar fragment greater than 2 mm, incomplete repositioning and age greater than 30 years. The risk of pulp canal obliteration after 10 years was 13% and for progressive root resorption was 13%. The type of splint and duration of splinting did not affect the risk for pulp necrosis [51].

There is also evidence that alveolar fractures treated more than 48 h after injury are at increased risk for pulp necrosis [49].

References

1. Anderson L, Petti S, Day P, Kenny K, Glendor U, Andreasen JO. Classification, epidemiology and etiology. In: Andreasen JO, Andreasen FM, Andersson L, editors. Textbook and color atlas of traumatic injuries to the teeth. 5th ed. Hoboken, NJ: Wiley-Blackwell; 2019. p. 252–94.
2. McTigue DJ. Managing traumatic injuries in the young permanent dentition. In: Nowak AJ, Christensen JR, Mabry TR, Townsend JA, Wells MH, editors. Pediatric dentistry infancy through adolescence. Philadelphia: Elsevier; 2019. p. 497–511.
3. Marcenes W, Murray S. Social deprivation and traumatic dental injuries among 14-year-old schoolchildren in Newham, London. Dent Traumatol. 2001;17:17–21.
4. Rhouma O, McMahon AD, Welbury R. Traumatic dental injury and social deprivation in five-year-old children in Scotland 1993-2007. Br Dent J. 2013;214:e26.
5. Da Rosa P, Rousseau MC, Edasseri A, Herderson M, Nicolau B. Investigating socioeconomic position in dental caries and traumatic dental injury among children in Quebec. Community Dent Health. 2017;34:226–33.
6. Bastos JV, Goulart EM, de Souza Cortes MI. Pulpal response to sensibility tests after traumatic dental injuries in permanent teeth. Dent Traumatol. 2014;30:188–92.
7. Jespersen JJ, Hellstein J, Williamson A, Johnson WT, Qian F. Evaluation of dental pulp sensibility tests in a clinical setting. J Endod. 2014;40:351–4.
8. Ahn SY, Kim D, Park SH. Efficacy of ultrasound Doppler flowmetry in assessing pulp vitality of traumatized teeth: a propensity score matching analysis. J Endod. 2018;44:379–83.
9. Andreasen JO, editor. The dental trauma guide. San Diego: International Association of Dental Traumatology; 2012.
10. Olsburgh S, Jacoby T, Krejci I. Crown fractures in the permanent dentition: pulpal and restorative considerations. Dent Traumatol. 2002;18:103–15.
11. Costa CA, Giro EM, do Nascimento AB, Teixeira HM, Hebling J. Short-term evaluation of the pulpo-dentin complex response to a resin-modified glass-ionomer cement and a bonding agent applied in deep cavities. Dent Mater. 2003;19:739–46.
12. Trope M, Barnett F, Sigurdsson A, Chivian N. The role of endodontics after dental traumatic injuries. In: Hargreaves KM, Berman LH, editors. Cohen's pathways of the pulp. 11th ed. St. Louis: Elsevier; 2016. p. 758–92.
13. DiAngelis AJ, Andreasen JO, Ebeleseder KA, Kenny DJ, Trope M, Sigurdsson A, Andersson L, Bourguignon C, Flores MT, Hicks ML, Lenzi AR, Malmgren B, Moule AJ, Pohl Y, Tsukiboshi M. Guidelines for the management of traumatic dental injuries: 1. Fractures and luxations of permanent teeth. Dent Traumatol. 2012;28:2–12.
14. Velan E. Restorative dentistry for the adolescent. In: Nowak AJ, Christensen JR, Mabry TR, Townsend JA, Wells MH, editors. Pediatric dentistry infancy through adolescence. Philadelphia: Elsevier; 2019. p. 598–609.

15. Andreasen FM, Noren JG, Andreasen JO, Engelhardtsen S, Lindh-Stromberg U. Long-term survival of fragment bonding in the treatment of fractured crowns: a multicenter clinical study. Quintessence Int. 1995;26:669–81.
16. Yilmaz Y, Guler C, Sahin H, Eyuboglu O. Evaluation of tooth-fragment reattachment: a clinical and laboratory study. Dent Traumatol. 2010;26:308–14.
17. Garcia FCP, Poubel DLN, Almeida JCF, Toledo IP, Poi WR, Guerra ENS, Rezende LVML. Tooth fragment reattachment techniques-a systematic review. Dent Traumatol. 2018;34:135–43.
18. Cvek M, Cleaton-Jones PE, Austin JC, Andreasen JO. Pulp reactions to exposure after experimental crown fractures in adult monkeys. J Endod. 1982;8:391–7.
19. He Y, Gan Y, Lu J, Feng Q, Wang H, Guan H, Jiang Q. Pulpal tissue inflammatory reactions after experimental pulpal exposure in mice. J Endod. 2017;43:90–5.
20. Parirokh M, Torabinejad M, Dummer PMH. Mineral trioxide aggregate and other bioactive endodontic cements: an updated overview - part I: vital pulp therapy. Int Endod J. 2018;51:177–205.
21. Kaur M, Singh H, Dhillon JS, Batra M, Saini M. MTA versus biodentine: review of literature with a comparative analysis. J Clin Diagn Res. 2017;11:ZG01–5. https://doi.org/10.7860/JCDR/2017/25840.10374.
22. Cvek M, Abbott PV, Bakland LK, Heithersay GS. Management of trauma-related pulp disease and tooth resorption. In: Andreasen JO, Andreasen FM, Andersson L, editors. Textbook and color atlas of traumatic injuries to the teeth. 5th ed. Hoboken: Wiley-Blackwell; 2019. p. 648–717.
23. Ravn JJ. Follow-up study of permanent incisors with complicated crown fractures after acute trauma. Scand J Dent Res. 1982;90:363–72.
24. Wang G, Wang C, Qin M. Pulp prognosis following conservative pulp treatment in teeth with complicated crown fractures-a retrospective study. Dent Traumatol. 2017;33:255–60.
25. Cvek M. A clinical report on partial pulpotomy and capping with calcium hydroxide in permanent incisors with complicated crown fracture. J Endod. 1978;4:232–7.
26. Andreasen JO, Andreasen FM, Tsukiboshi M, Eichelsbacher F. Crown-root fracture. In: Andreasen JO, Andreasen FM, Andersson L, editors. Textbook and color atlas of traumatic injuries to the teeth. 5th ed. Hoboken: Wiley-Blackwell; 2019. p. 355–76.
27. Cohenca N, Silberman A. Contemporary imaging for the diagnosis and treatment of traumatic dental injuries: a review. Dent Traumatol. 2017;33:321–8.
28. De Castro MA, Poi WR, de Castro JC, Panzarini SR, Sonoda CK, Trevisan CL, Luvizuto ER. Crown and crown-root fractures: an evaluation of the treatment plans for management proposed by 154 specialists in restorative dentistry. Dent Traumatol. 2010;26:236–42.
29. Eichelsbacher F, Denner W, Klaiber B, Schlagenhauf U. Periodontal status of teeth with crown-root fractures: results two years after adhesive fragment reattachment. J Clin Periodontol. 2009;36:905–11.
30. Jardim Pdos S, Negri MR, Masotti AS. Rehabilitation to crown-root fracture by fragment reattachment with resin-modified glass ionomer cement and composite resin restoration. Dent Traumatol. 2010;26:186–90.
31. Heithersay GS. Combined endodontic-orthodontic treatment of transverse root fractures in the region of the alveolar crest. Oral Surg Oral Med Oral Pathol. 1973;36:404–15.
32. Wolfson EM, Seiden L. Combined endodontic-orthodontic treatment of subgingivally fractured teeth. J Can Dent Assoc. 1975;11:621–4.
33. Simon JHS, Kelly WH, Gordon DG, Ericksen GW. Extrusion of endodontically treated teeth. J Am Dent Assoc. 1978;97:17–23.
34. Fidel SR, Fidel-Junior RA, Sassone LM, Murad CF, Fidel RA. Clinical management of a complicated crown-root fracture: a case report. Braz Dent J. 2011;22:258–62.
35. O'Toole S, Garvey T, Hashem A. The multidisciplinary conservative management of a vital crown root fracture. Dent Update. 2013;40:584–6.
36. Wang J, Li M. Multidisciplinary treatment of a complicated crown-root fracture. Pediatr Dent. 2010;32:250–4.

37. Martins AV, Albuquerque RC, Lanza LD, Vilaca EL, Silva N, Moreira AN, da Silveira RR. Conservative treatment of a complicated crown-root fracture using adhesive fragment reattachment and composite resin restoration: two year follow-up. Oper Dent. 2018;43:E102–9.
38. Tegsjo U, Valerius-Olsson H, Olgart K. Intra-alveolar transplantation of teeth with cervical root fractures. Swed Dent J. 1978;2:73–82.
39. Tegsjo U, Valerius-Olsson H, Frykholm A, Olgart K. Clinical evaluation of intra-alveolar transplantation of teeth with cervical root fractures. Swed Dent J. 1987;11:235–50.
40. Kahnberg KE. Intra-alveolar transplantation. I. A 10-year follow-up of a method for surgical extrusion of root fractured teeth. Swed Dent J. 1996;20:165–72.
41. Warfvinge J, Kahnberg KE. Intraalveolar transplantation of teeth. IV. Endodontic considerations. Swed Dent J. 1989;13:229–33.
42. Malmgren B, Cvek M, Lundberg M, Frykholm A. Surgical treatment of ankylosed and infrapositioned reimplanted incisors in adolescents. Scand J Dent Res. 1984;92:391–9.
43. Elkhadem A, Mickan S, Richards D. Adverse events of surgical extrusion in treatment for crown-root and cervical root fractures: a systematic review of case series/reports. Dent Traumatol. 2014;30:1–14.
44. Das B, Muthu MS. Surgical extrusion as a treatment option for crown-root fracture in permanent anterior teeth: a systematic review. Dent Traumatol. 2013;29:423–31.
45. Andreasen FM, Andreasen JO, Tsilingaridis G. Root fractures. In: Andreasen JO, Andreasen FM, Andersson L, editors. Textbook and color atlas of traumatic injuries to the teeth. 5th ed. Hoboken: Wiley-Blackwell; 2019. p. 377–412.
46. Bender IB, Freedland JB. Clinical considerations in the diagnosis and treatment of intra-alveolar root fractures. J Am Dent Assoc. 1983;107:595–600.
47. Andreasen FM. Pulpal healing after luxation injuries and root fracture in the permanent dentition. Endod Dent Traumatol. 1989;5:111–31.
48. Andreasen JO, Ahrensburg SS, Tsilingaridis G. Root fractures: the influence of type of healing and location of fracture on tooth survival rates - an analysis of 492 cases. Dent Traumatol. 2012;28:404–9.
49. Andreasen JO, Lauridsen E. Injuries to the supporting bone. In: Andreasen JO, Andreasen FM, Andersson L, editors. Textbook and color atlas of traumatic injuries to the teeth. 5th ed. Hoboken: Wiley-Blackwell; 2019. p. 529–55.
50. Andreasen JO, Lauridsen E. Alveolar process fractures in the permanent dentition. Part 1. Etiology and clinical characteristics. A retrospective analysis of 299 cases involving 815 teeth. Dent Traumatol. 2015;31:442–7.
51. Lauridsen E, Gerds T, Andreasen JO. Alveolar process fractures in the permanent dentition. Part 2. The risk of healing complications in teeth involved in an alveolar process fracture. Dent Traumatol. 2016;32:128–39.

Permanent Tooth Luxation Injuries

Luxation injuries range from very mild, as in the case of a concussion of the tooth, to very severe when the tooth is avulsed completely out of the socket. Between these entities there are injuries that dislodge teeth in such a way that the supporting bone may also sustain an injury. In each type of trauma, it is essential to determine the full extent of injury to the tooth, the pulp, the periodontium, supporting bone, and any other hard or soft tissue of the body. Andreasen et al. estimate that 15–61% of dental traumatic injuries to permanent teeth are due to luxation injuries [1]. In the permanent and mixed dentitions, the etiology of a traumatic injury is most likely to be from a fall or from a sports-related injury. In this age group, there is still a concern for intentional injuries, so this should always be kept in mind and investigated further if suspicions arise regarding the cause of an injury.

7.1 Concussion

Concussion is the mildest of dental injuries of permanent teeth. The tooth is not mobile and is not displaced. It is sensitive to pressure or percussion. There is no evidence of sulcular bleeding, and the tooth responds positively to sensibility testing. Radiographic evaluation is indicated to establish a baseline and to rule out a root fracture. This will also show the presence of any dislocations of the tooth in the socket. A lack of dislocation, history of traumatic injury, and sensitivity to percussion is a confirmation of the diagnosis of concussion. It is recommended to use a film holder to minimize errors and to have consistent angulation at future follow-up appointments [2].

7.1.1 Treatment Recommendations

No treatment is indicated unless other teeth have sustained more extensive trauma. Since the symptoms are minimal, patients with this type of injury may not present to the dentist for evaluation at the time of the trauma. If the patient complains of

© Springer Nature Switzerland AG 2020

R. L. Slayton, E. A. Palmer, *Traumatic Dental Injuries in Children*,

https://doi.org/10.1007/978-3-030-25793-4_7

discomfort, Tylenol or ibuprofen can be recommended. Avoiding additional trauma to the affected tooth or teeth is recommended. Following a soft food diet for 1 week and maintaining good oral hygiene will aid in the healing process.

7.1.2   Follow-Up

It is recommended that the patient be seen for clinical and radiographic examination at 4 weeks, 6–8 weeks, and 1 year [3]. At these visits, sensibility testing should also be recorded to monitor changes and risks for pulp necrosis.

7.1.3   Prognosis

The prognosis is expected to be excellent and is dependent on the maturity of the tooth at the time of the injury. Pulp necrosis and root resorption are rare [4]. In the few cases with concussion injuries that demonstrated pulp necrosis in Andreasen and Pedersen's study, all had mature root apices. Of the 120 teeth with mature apices and a concussion injury, 5 (4.1%) developed pulp necrosis [4]. In another study of teeth with combination injuries, Lauridsen et al. [5] found that 3.5% of mature teeth with concussion injuries alone had pulp necrosis within the first year. Mature teeth with concussion injuries and uncomplicated crown fractures had an 11% risk for pulp necrosis within the first year [5]. Teeth with concussion and uncomplicated crown fractures with negative sensibility tests at the time of injury had a 55% risk for pulp necrosis at the end of 1 year [5]. It is not unusual for teeth to have more than one type of injury after a traumatic accident. It is important to understand the additional risk related to concomitant injuries so patients and families can be informed and appropriate follow-up is provided.

Periodontal healing complications are very low for teeth with concussion injuries. In a longitudinal study by Hermann et al. [6], 469 permanent teeth with concussion injury were evaluated. There were no healing complications reported in teeth with immature apices. Among teeth with mature apices, the risk of repair-related resorption was 3.2% and the risk of marginal bone loss was 0.7%. There were no cases that demonstrated infection-related resorption or replacement resorption [6]. The majority of patients in this study were under 20 years of age but the study also included individuals over 20 years.

7.2   Subluxation

Subluxation is a traumatic injury to the tooth or teeth that results in detectable mobility without displacement. Presence of bleeding around the gingival sulcus in addition to radiographic evaluation confirms the diagnosis (Fig. 7.1). The tooth is sensitive to touch and percussion. A radiograph is made to rule out a root fracture, assess the root development, and establish a baseline. Pulp sensibility testing should be done and it may be negative initially. This is a sign of transient pulpal injury. A positive test is

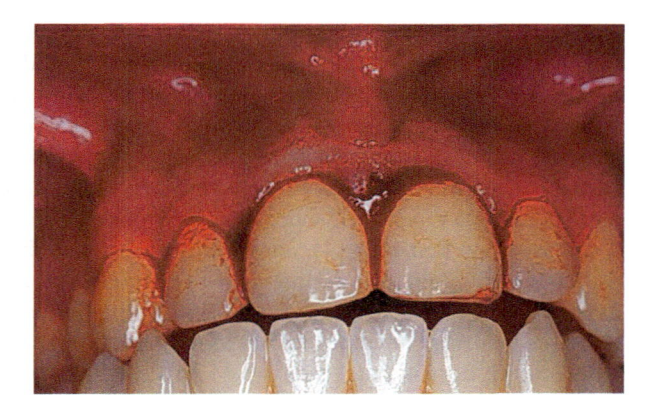

Fig. 7.1 Subluxation of maxillary permanent incisors. Sulcular bleeding is evident and the teeth are sensitive to touch and percussion

likely to be seen about half of the time. It is important to remember that although a negative test at the time of injury is not a definitive diagnosis of pulpal health, it has been shown to indicate a risk for pulpal necrosis in the future [2, 7].

7.2.1 Treatment Recommendations

There is usually no need for treatment. If the slight mobility is uncomfortable for the patient, a flexible splint can be placed for 2 weeks. As with concussion injuries, since the symptoms are minimal, patients with this type of injury may not present to the dentist for evaluation at the time of the trauma. It is important to document the history of traumatic injuries when patients are seen for routine care. Even if the patient wasn't seen at the time of the injury, the history of trauma should signal the need for a follow-up plan for the affected teeth. If the patient complains of discomfort, acetaminophen or ibuprofen can be recommended. Avoiding additional trauma to the affected tooth or teeth is recommended. Following a soft food diet for 1 week and maintaining good oral hygiene will aid in the healing process [3].

7.2.2 Follow-Up

The patient should be seen for clinical and radiographic examination at 2 weeks, 4 weeks, 6–8 weeks and 1 year [3]. If a splint was placed, it should be removed at 2 weeks. Sensibility tests should be performed at each follow-up visit to monitor for changes and pulp necrosis.

7.2.3 Prognosis

There is limited data regarding the prognosis for immature teeth following a subluxation injury. The most common sequelae for mature teeth with a subluxation injury are pulp necrosis and pulp obliteration. In the cases with subluxation injuries that demonstrated pulp necrosis in Andreasen and Pedersen's study, all had mature root apices [4]. Of the 93 teeth with mature apices and a subluxation injury, 14 (15%) developed pulp necrosis [4]. In another study of teeth with combination injuries, Lauridsen et al. [8] found some risk for pulp necrosis in both immature and mature teeth. In immature teeth with no concomitant crown fracture, none developed pulp necrosis. This is consistent with the findings from Andreasen and Pedersen [4]. However, immature teeth with subluxation injuries and concomitant enamel-dentin crown fracture had a 25% risk for pulp necrosis in the first year. For immature teeth with subluxation and enamel-dentin crown fractures that responded negatively to pulp sensibility tests at the initial visit, the risk for pulp necrosis at 1 year was 57.1% [8]. As with concussion injuries, the risk for pulp necrosis was greater in teeth with mature apices. The authors reported that 12.5% of mature teeth with subluxation injuries alone had pulp necrosis within the first year [8]. Mature teeth with subluxation injuries and uncomplicated enamel-dentin crown fractures had a 54.8% risk for pulp necrosis within the first year [8]. Teeth with subluxation and uncomplicated crown fractures with negative sensibility tests at the time of injury had an 86.7% risk for pulp necrosis at the end of 1 year [8]. It is not unusual for teeth to have more than one type of injury after a traumatic event. It is important to understand the additional risk related to concomitant injuries so patients and families can be informed and appropriate follow-up is provided.

Periodontal healing complications are very low for teeth with subluxation injuries. In a longitudinal study by Hermann et al. [6], 404 permanent teeth with subluxation injury were evaluated. There was a 1.7% risk for infection-related resorption in teeth with immature apices after 3 years. Among teeth with mature apices, the risk of repair-related resorption was 3.6% and the risk of marginal bone loss was 0.6%. The risk for infection-related resorption and replacement-related resorption was 0.6% [6]. The majority of patients in this study were under 20 years of age but the study also included individuals over 20 years.

7.3   Lateral Luxation

Estimates of the frequency of lateral luxation injuries in children and adolescents vary. One study found that lateral luxations accounted for 11% of traumatized permanent teeth [9]. This injury involves the displacement of the tooth in a palatal or labial direction and generally involves fracture of the alveolar bone from the displacement of the root (Figs. 7.2a–c and 7.3a–c). This results in severance of the neurovascular supply and periodontal ligament. The diagnosis is made from a clinical and radiographic evaluation. The tooth is often not mobile but may be interfering with normal occlusion. It may be possible to feel the apex of the luxated tooth at the point of penetration through the buccal plate. When the tooth root is locked in the fractured portion of the alveolus, percussion tests will be similar to that for intruded teeth.

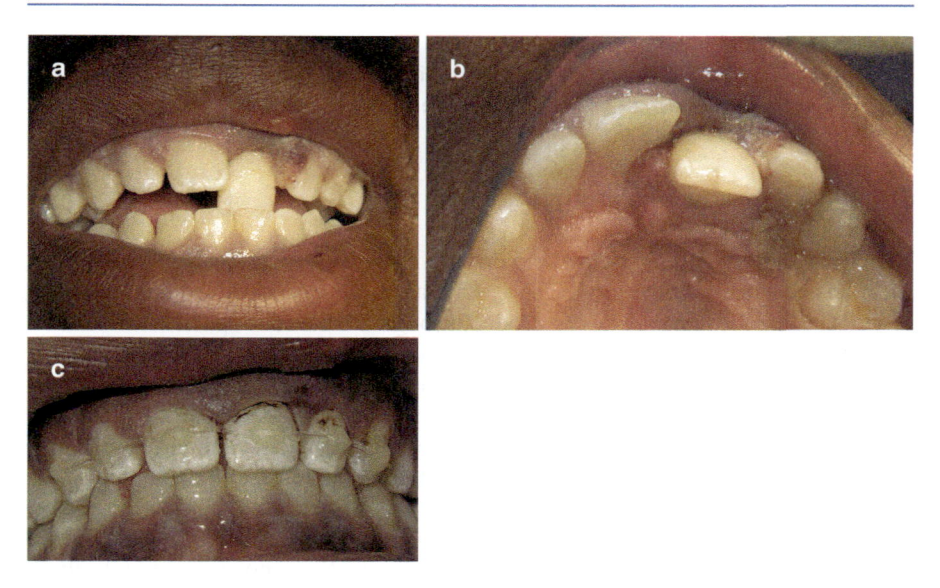

Fig. 7.2 Frontal (**a**) and occlusal (**b**) view of a lateral luxation of maxillary left central incisor interfering with occlusion. The tooth was repositioned and splinted with monofilament (**c**)

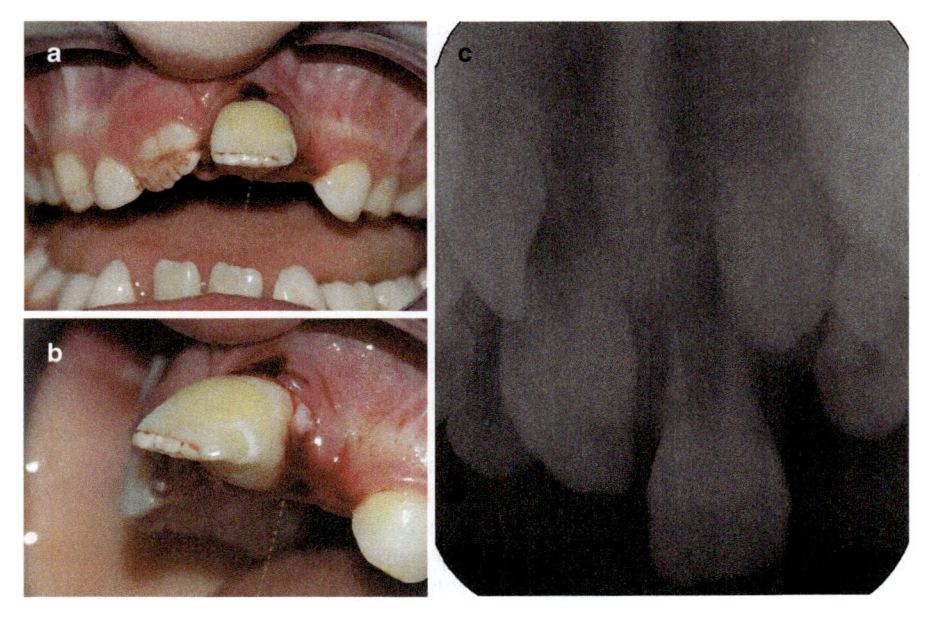

Fig. 7.3 Frontal (**a**) and lateral (**b**) view of a lateral luxation of a maxillary left central incisor including fracture of the alveolar bone. In the radiograph (**c**), it appears that the tooth is extruded. (Courtesy of Dr. Monica Cipes)

Radiographically, a laterally luxated tooth will show an increase in apical periodontal space when the tooth is displaced labially (Fig. 7.3c). This will depend on the exposure and direction of the central beam of the X-ray head [10].

7.3.1   Treatment Recommendations

The tooth should be repositioned either with forceps or finger pressure following local anesthesia administration. The tooth may need to be extruded slightly prior to repositioning if the apex has protruded through the buccal or palatal bone creating a bony lock. This should be attempted initially by putting digital pressure in the vicinity of the root tip in the sulcular fold. If digital pressure is not adequate to reposition the tooth, forceps can be used to gently extrude the tooth slightly to unlock the root from the bone. After repositioning, the palatal and labial plates of the alveolar bone should be compressed together. This will facilitate healing [10]. Once the tooth is repositioned, a flexible splint is placed for 4 weeks (Fig. 7.2c). A radiograph should be made to verify the position and to use as a comparison in the future. Any soft tissue injuries should be sutured after repositioning and splinting the teeth.

If there is a delay in treating the patient, it may be difficult to reposition the luxated tooth. If it is not interfering with occlusion, there are some situations where the tooth can be permitted to spontaneously reposition. When there is occlusal interference, repositioning the tooth to eliminate this interference is important. In some cases, orthodontic repositioning can be done in combination with splinting.

Children and adolescents with complex medical conditions, anxiety or developmental disabilities may not be able to cooperate for treatment in the traditional dental setting. In these cases, treatment in a hospital operating room under general anesthesia may be indicated. Sedation in the office or in an emergency room is an option for some children if it can be performed safely.

7.3.2   Follow-Up

The IADT Trauma guidelines recommend clinical and radiographic examination at 2 weeks, 4 weeks, 6–8 weeks, 6 months, and annually for 5 years [3]. The splint should be removed at 4 weeks. For immature teeth, radiographs should show continuing root development. For mature teeth, regular evaluation for pulp vitality should be done. When pulp necrosis occurs, it is most likely to occur within the first year and is much more likely if there is a concomitant crown fracture.

It should be emphasized that traumatized teeth may have a negative response to sensibility testing for up to 3 months after the injury. In addition, the phenomenon known as transient apical breakdown (TAB) can create a diagnostic challenge that could lead to a decision to initiate endodontic therapy prematurely. Andreasen et al. describe this as internal resorption at the apices of mature teeth in combination with discoloration of the clinical crown and temporary loss of pulpal sensibility [10]. It is thought to be part of the pulpal healing process that permits new blood vessels and nerves to become established in the pulp. This condition has been shown to return to normal and does not require root canal treatment. The incidence of TAB is low. Andreasen [13] identified this condition in 4.2% of 637 cases of permanent tooth luxations. More recently, Cohenca et al, presented a case of a 15-year-old girl with this diagnosis [14]. Many of the diagnostic signs suggested that root canal treatment was indicated: discoloration of the crown, apical radiolucency, and lack of response to sensibility testing. However, the tooth was asymptomatic to percussion and palpation. At a subsequent evaluation, the tooth responded to cold and electric pulp testing and there were radiographic signs of healing. The authors make the point that in cases where the diagnosis is unclear and the patient and family can be counted on to follow-up with care, it is reasonable to "watch and wait" rather than initiate root canal treatment. However, since the literature has documented the relatively high rates of pulp necrosis in mature permanent tooth luxations, the decision to initiate endodontic therapy may be appropriate, especially when the family has a history of non-compliance with recommendations [14]. Although TAB is a relatively uncommon finding, the opportunity for misdiagnosis exists and it is important to be aware of this phenomenon to avoid unnecessary endodontic treatment.

7.3.3 Prognosis

There is limited data for the prognosis of immature teeth with luxation injuries. For mature teeth, the most common sequelae are pulp necrosis and pulpal obliteration. Andreasen and Pedersen found that 9% of immature teeth and 77% of mature teeth became necrotic after lateral luxation injuries [4]. Other complications included pulp canal obliteration (28% of teeth affected) and root resorption (27% of teeth affected). In a study that was limited to adolescent patients, Nikoui et al. evaluated the healing outcomes for 58 teeth from 42 patients with laterally luxated permanent maxillary incisors [11]. Pulp necrosis was seen in 40% of the teeth. The frequency of pulp canal obliteration was also 40% and there was no increased risk based on tooth maturity [11]. Most cases with pulp necrosis occurred in the first year after the injury in both studies. Lauridsen et al. evaluated the risk for pulp necrosis in 179 teeth with lateral luxation with or without a concomitant crown fracture [12]. The teeth were further evaluated based on the root development. The risk of pulp necrosis in immature teeth with no crown fracture was 4.7% and this increased to 40% if there was a concomitant uncomplicated crown fracture [12]. For mature teeth, the risk of pulp necrosis was 65.1% for luxation alone and 93% when there was a concomitant uncomplicated crown fracture [12]. In this study, the authors found that a negative response to sensibility testing at the initial examination was not associated with subsequent pulp necrosis [12].

7.4   Extrusive Luxation

Extrusive luxation describes the partial displacement of a tooth out of the socket. The socket remains intact and there is no lateral displacement (Fig. 7.4a). Diagnosis is made from clinical and radiographic findings. A radiograph is made to rule out a root fracture, to assess the degree of root development, and to establish a baseline. The tooth will be tender and mobile. Extrusive luxation injuries cause rupture of the neurovascular supply to the pulp and damage to the periodontal ligament fibers [10]. The clinical and radiographic appearance will be elongation of the tooth. Bleeding will be present from the periodontal ligament and mobility will be evident. Sensitivity to percussion is expected. At the initial visit, sensibility tests are likely to be negative, however, a positive response at this initial visit indicates a reduced risk of pulp necrosis later [7].

The frequency of extrusive luxation was found to be 7% in one study that included adults and 1.3% in a study limited to 7–18-year olds [9, 15]. In a trauma center affiliated with a hospital in the U.S., 4% of the traumatic injuries treated at the hospital were extrusive injuries of permanent teeth [16].

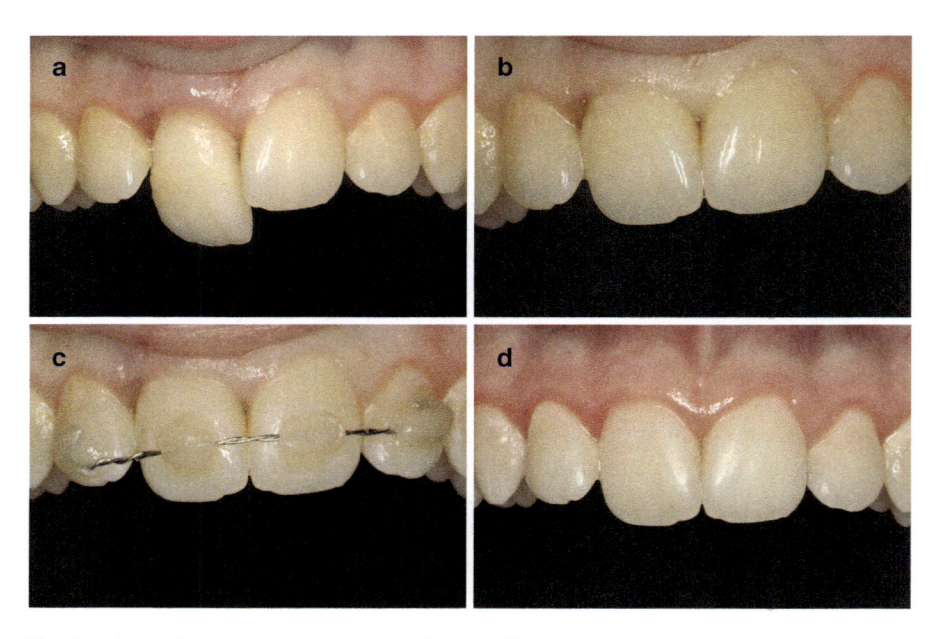

Fig. 7.4 Extrusive luxation of permanent right maxillary central incisor (**a**). The tooth was repositioned (**b**) and splinted with a flexible archwire (**c**). At the follow-up appointment, the tooth was asymptomatic with no evidence of ankylosis (**d**). (Courtesy of Dr. Simon Jenn-Yih Lin)

7.4.1 Treatment Recommendations

After cleansing the exposed root surface, digital pressure is used to reposition the tooth in the socket (Fig. 7.4b). Local anesthesia may not be necessary. Once the tooth is repositioned, a flexible splint is placed for 2 weeks (Fig. 7.4c). If there has been a delay in treatment following the injury, the clot in the socket may make repositioning difficult. In this case, orthodontic repositioning may be necessary [7].

7.4.2 Follow-Up

Immature teeth should be monitored for root development as a sign of continued pulp vitality. Mature teeth are monitored for pulp vitality and absence of pathologic changes. Clinical and radiographic examinations should be done at 2 weeks when the splint is removed and then at 4 weeks, 6–8 weeks, 6 months, 1 year and yearly for 5 years [3, 7].

Findings that indicate that healing is occurring include:

- The tooth is asymptomatic—no pain to percussion or palpation
- Radiographic signs of healed periodontium—no periapical radiolucency
- Positive response to pulp testing—false negative is possible up to 3 months
- Normal position of marginal bone
- Continued root development—apices closing, pulp canal walls thickening

Findings that indicate non-healing:

- Tooth is symptomatic—sensitive to percussion and/or palpation
- Negative response to pulp testing—false negative is possible up to 3 months
- Breakdown of marginal bone
- External inflammatory root resorption

7.4.3 Prognosis

There is limited data regarding the prognosis for immature teeth with extrusive luxation injuries. The most common sequelae for mature teeth with extrusive luxation injuries are pulp necrosis and pulpal obliteration. Andreasen and Pedersen [4] found that 9% of immature teeth with extrusive luxation developed pulp necrosis and 55% of teeth with closed apices developed pulp necrosis. Pulp canal obliteration was more common in teeth with an open apex (61%) than when the apex was closed (20%) [4]. In a study of extrusive luxation and concomitant crown fractures, Lauridsen et al. found that the risk of pulp necrosis for teeth with immature apices and no crown fracture was 5.9% after 1 year [12]. In this sample, none of the extruded teeth with immature apices developed pulp necrosis and there was no significant difference between the groups with or without crown fracture. For mature teeth with extrusive luxation, there was no statistically significant difference for the risk of pulp necrosis between those with and without concomitant crown fracture.

The risk without crown fracture was 56.5% and the risk with crown fracture was 76.5% [12]. Healing complications related to the periodontium are relatively low for extrusive luxation injuries. In a study of 82 permanent teeth with extrusive luxation, Hermann et al. [17] reported that no teeth developed ankylosis-related resorption and that infection-related resorption occurred in 2.4% of immature teeth [17]. Periodontal healing complications were more frequent in teeth with mature apices. In mature teeth, 15.6% developed repair-related resorption, 5.1% had infection-related resorption, and 17.5% demonstrated marginal bone loss [17].

7.5　Intrusion

Intrusive luxation is the vertical displacement of a tooth into the socket. This results in a fracture of the alveolar socket and damage to the periodontal ligament. Diagnosis is made from clinical and radiographic findings (Fig. 7.5a–d). Severe intrusion may

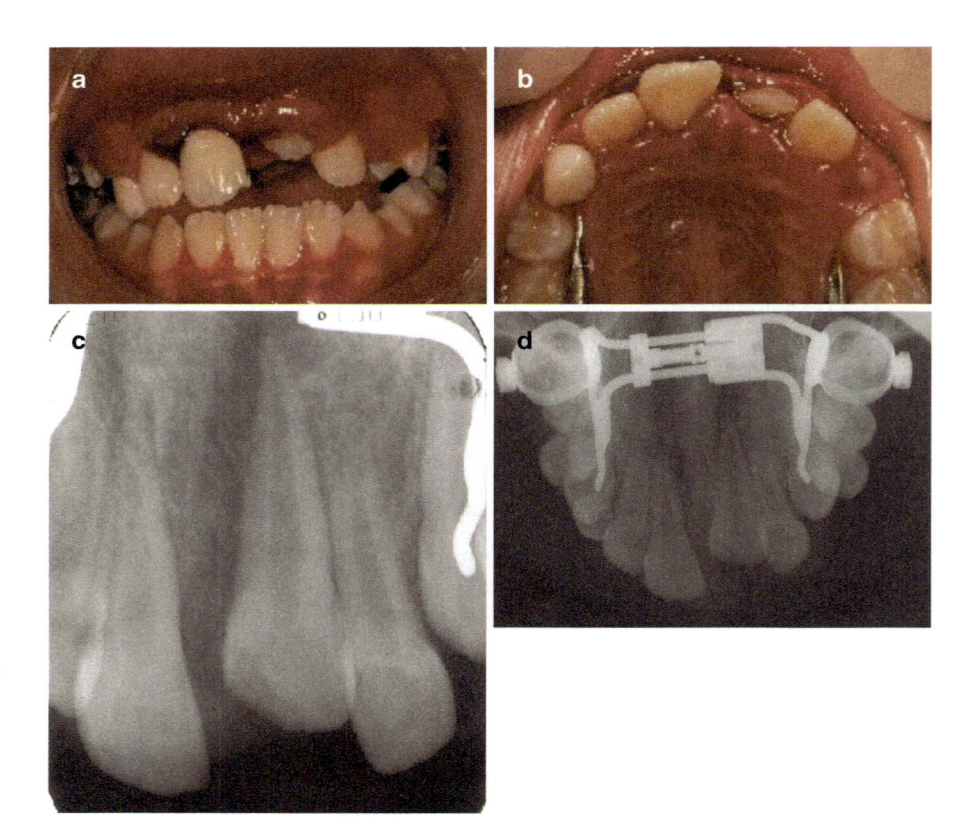

Fig. 7.5 Frontal (**a**) and occlusal (**b**) view of a left central incisor with severe intrusion. The tooth has a closed apex (**c**). A palatal expansion appliance is in place as a result of ongoing orthodontic treatment (**d**). (Courtesy of Dr. Nestor Cohenca)

appear clinically the same as avulsion and should be confirmed with a radiograph. The intruded tooth is not usually mobile. One or more radiographs are made to assess the extent of the intrusion, rule out root fracture, and provide a baseline. Depending on the extent of the intrusion, a lateral external radiograph may be indicated to rule out penetration of the root into the floor of the nasal cavity. The periodontal ligament may or may not be visible radiographically [18].

If part of the crown is still visible, percussion testing will produce a high metallic sound, similar to ankylosed teeth. This may help to distinguish between a partially erupted tooth and an intruded tooth [7, 18]. It is likely that sensibility tests will be negative at the time of the injury. Concomitant injuries such as lateral luxation and crown fracture are also possible and should be managed as described previously.

Published reports document a frequency of 0.3–2.4% in the permanent dentition [18]. In a study of 216 intruded permanent teeth over a 50-year period, Andreasen et al. found that this type of injury happened most frequently in children between 6 and 12 years of age and more often in boys than girls. In 33.5% of the cases, the injury was limited to the intrusion while 60.5% of the time, there was a concomitant crown fracture [19]. Many of the longitudinal studies of traumatic dental injuries are based in Copenhagen and Sweden, where there are long standing trauma centers. One study in the U.S. evaluated traumatic dental injuries treated at a Children's Hospital and reported similar findings to those of Andreasen et al. regarding the frequency of intrusive luxation injuries. In the study by Ziegler of 1218 teeth with traumatic dental injuries, 4% were intrusive luxation injuries and the most common age for this injury was between 6 and 10 years [16].

7.5.1 Treatment Recommendations

Andreasen et al. [18] describe three current treatment modalities for intruded permanent teeth. The choice of treatment depends on the extent of the intrusion and the degree of root development. Immature teeth with intrusion less than 7 mm should be allowed to re-erupt spontaneously. It is expected to take about 6 months for an intruded permanent tooth to fully re-erupt. During this time, the tooth should be monitored for signs of movement, continued root development or pulp necrosis. Endodontic treatment should be initiated if there are signs of necrosis. After 1 month, if the tooth is not re-erupting or if there are signs of ankylosis, orthodontic repositioning should be initiated. For immature teeth with intrusion greater than 7 mm either surgical or orthodontic repositioning should be done [3, 7, 18].

For mature teeth, spontaneous re-eruption is only recommended for mild intrusion (less than 3 mm). For moderate intrusions between 3 and 7 mm, surgical or orthodontic repositioning is recommended and for severe intrusion (greater than 7 mm), surgical repositioning is recommended. In addition, endodontic therapy should be initiated between 3 and 4 weeks following the trauma. A splint is placed for 4 weeks once repositioning is complete [3, 7, 18].

When orthodontic repositioning is the treatment of choice, this can be initiated at the initial visit or a few days later (Fig. 7.6a–c). In cases of severe intrusion, it may

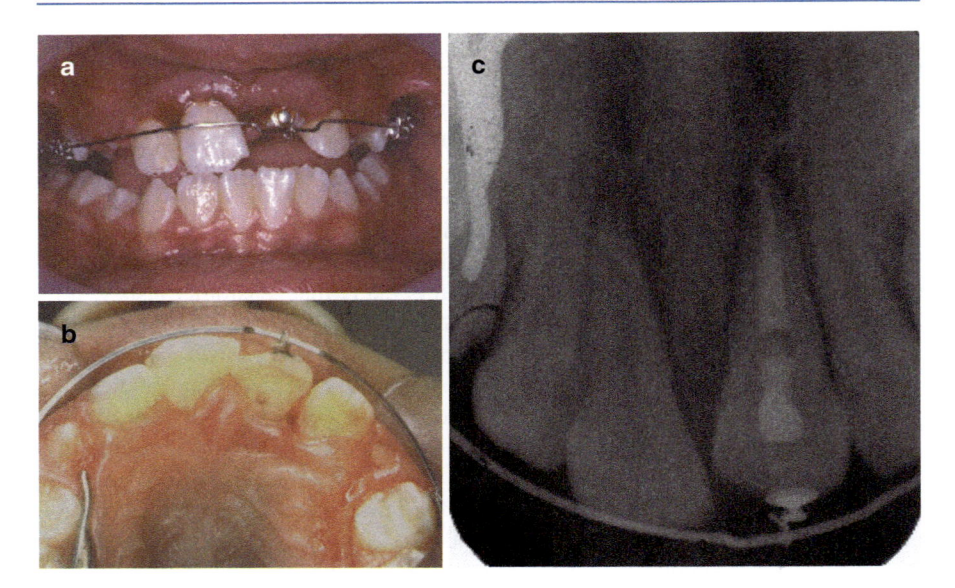

Fig. 7.6 Orthodontic extrusion (**a**) was initiated and endodontic treatment completed once the tooth was extruded enough to achieve good isolation (**b**). A post-endo radiograph was made as a baseline (**c**). (Courtesy of Dr. Nestor Cohenca)

be necessary to reposition the tooth partially using forceps so that there is enough exposed tooth structure to bond to. With mature teeth, adequate exposure should be accomplished within 3–4 weeks so that endodontic treatment can be initiated. When the intruded tooth has been repositioned and the splint removed, a final restoration can be placed (Fig. 7.7a, b).

Surgical repositioning involves using forceps to move the intruded tooth into its normal position immediately. It is recommended that the forceps engage the proximal surfaces of the tooth rather than facial and palatal surfaces. Once in position, digital pressure is used to reposition the facial and palatal bone and a splint is placed for 4–8 weeks [7, 18]. When multiple teeth are injured or in cases of the mixed dentition, it may be necessary to extend the splint to the permanent molars to achieve adequate stability.

As with many traumatic dental injuries and their treatment, there is a lack of high-quality, long-term clinical trials with large numbers of patients to adequately evaluate the various treatment options. Retrospective studies provide some guidance and have informed the current treatment guidelines [3]. Table 7.1 summarizes the current recommendations for treatment of intruded permanent teeth based on root development and extent of intrusion [7].

7.5.2 Follow-Up

Clinical and radiographic examination at 4 weeks, 6–8 weeks, 6 months, and annually for 5 years. Splint removal at 4 weeks for orthodontic repositioning and at 6–8

Fig. 7.7 Following completion of the extrusion (**a**), the fractured incisal edge is restored (**b**). (Courtesy of Dr. Nestor Cohenca)

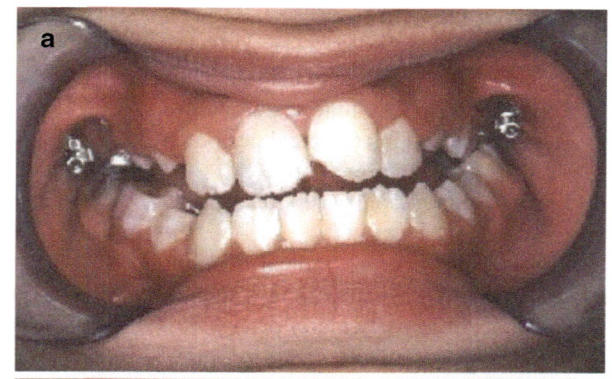

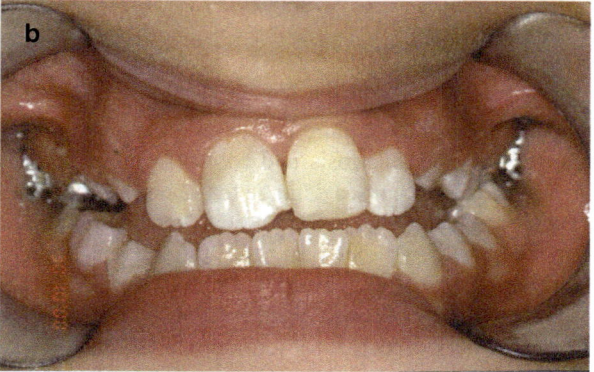

Table 7.1 Duration of splinting for each type of injury

Type of injury	Splint duration
Concussion	None
Subluxation	None
Lateral luxation	4 weeks
Extrusive luxation	2 weeks
Intrusion	
Surgical reposition	6–8 weeks
Orthodontic reposition	4 weeks

weeks for surgical repositioning [3]. Once the tooth extrusion is complete, a composite restoration is done.

Findings that indicate that healing is occurring include:

- Tooth is returning to original position relative to non-intruded tooth
- The tooth is asymptomatic—no pain to percussion or palpation
- Radiographic signs of intact lamina dura
- Positive response to pulp testing—false negative is possible up to 3 months
- Continued root development—apices closing, pulp canal walls thickening

Findings that indicate non-healing:

- Tooth has not returned to original position
- Tooth has ankylotic tone to percussion
- Radiographic signs of apical periodontitis
- Breakdown of marginal bone
- External inflammatory root resorption

Signs of pulp necrosis indicate that endodontic therapy should be initiated. If the tooth is ankylosed, treatment may include decoronation or extraction. Ankylosis in a growing child is particularly problematic and should be addressed in a timely way. This is discussed in more detail in Chap. 9.

7.5.3 Prognosis

Intruded teeth with mature apices are at significant risk for pulp necrosis and may also experience ankylosis and root resorption. This type of injury is considered severe because it causes damage to the bone within the alveolar socket, the gingival attachment, and the periodontal ligament. In immature teeth, there can also be damage to Hertwig's epithelial root sheath. The long-term prognosis for intruded permanent teeth is generally considered to be poor [18].

When the apex is open, there is still a chance for revascularization and this should be the primary objective for immature teeth.

A number of longitudinal retrospective studies have documented the healing outcomes for intruded permanent teeth based on severity of intrusion, root maturity, and type of treatment. Tsilingaridis et al, reported on a study of 60 intruded permanent teeth with three different treatment protocols [20]. Of these teeth, 17 were permitted to spontaneously re-erupt, 12 teeth were managed using orthodontic repositioning, and the remaining 31 teeth were repositioned surgically. The best healing outcomes were for immature teeth that were allowed to re-erupt spontaneously. The worst outcomes were for teeth that were surgically repositioned, but these were also teeth that were mature and had the most severe intrusion. Ankylosis was the most severe healing complication and led to the loss of 11 teeth [20]. A more recent study combined data from three separate studies of intruded permanent teeth. This allowed the authors to compare outcomes for three different treatment modalities in a pool of 230 intruded teeth. In this study, pulp necrosis occurred in 75% of the teeth and replacement resorption in 22%. The likelihood of both pulp necrosis and replacement resorption increased with the severity of intrusion. None of the teeth with mild intrusion developed replacement resorption [21].

Andreasen et al. [18] summarized clinical studies that reported the prognosis for intruded permanent teeth. In the 12 studies that were published over a 35-year period, pulp necrosis occurred in a range of 41–96% of teeth, root resorption in a range of 31–80% of teeth and loss of marginal bone in a range of 6–48% of teeth. Immature teeth that are allowed to re-erupt spontaneously have the least number of healing complications. However, long-term survival for intruded permanent teeth in general, is poor. Andreasen et al. report that after 15 years, regardless of the level of root development, 30% of intruded teeth are lost [18].

References

1. Andreasen FM, Andreasen JO, Lauridsen E. Luxation injuries of permanent teeth: general findings. In: Andreasen JO, Andreasen FM, Andersson L, editors. Textbook and color atlas of traumatic injuries to the teeth. 5th ed. Hoboken: Wiley-Blackwell; 2019. p. 413–42.
2. Andreasen FM, Lauridsen E, Andreasen JO. Concussion and subluxation. In: Andreasen JO, Andreasen FM, Andersson L, editors. Textbook and color atlas of traumatic injuries to the teeth. 5th ed. Hoboken: Wiley-Blackwell; 2019. p. 443–9.
3. DiAngelis AJ, Andreasen JO, Ebeleseder KA, Kenny DJ, Trope M, Sigurdsson A, Andersson L, Bourguignon C, Flores MT, Hicks ML, Lenzi AR, Malmgren B, Moule AJ, Pohl Y, Tsukiboshi M. Guidelines for the management of traumatic dental injuries: 1. Fractures and luxations of permanent teeth. Dent Traumatol. 2012;28:2–12.
4. Andreasen FM, Pedersen BV. Prognosis of luxated permanent teeth: the development of pulp necrosis. Endod Dent Traumatol. 1985;1:207–20.
5. Lauridsen E, Hermann NV, Gerds TA, Ahrensburg SS, Kreiborg S, Andreasen JO. Combination injuries I. The risk of pulp necrosis in permanent teeth with concussion injuries and concomitant crown fractures. Dent Traumatol. 2012;28:364–70.
6. Hermann NV, Lauridsen E, Ahrensburg SS, Gerds TA, Andreasen JO. Periodontal healing complications following concussion and subluxation injuries in the permanent dentition: a longitudinal cohort study. Dent Traumatol. 2012;28:386–93.
7. Andreasen JO, editor. The dental trauma guide. San Diego: International Association of Dental Traumatology; 2012.
8. Lauridsen E, Hermann NV, Gerds TA, Ahrensburg SS, Kreiborg S, Andreasen JO. Combination injuries 2. The risk of pulp necrosis in permanent teeth with subluxation injuries and concomitant crown fractures. Dent Traumatol. 2012;28:371–8.
9. Borum MK, Andreasen JO. Therapeutic and economic implications of traumatic dental injuries in Denmark; an estimate based on 7549 patients treated at a major trauma centre. Int J Paediatr Dent. 2001;11:249–58.
10. Andreasen FM, Lauridsen E, Andreasen JO. Extrusive luxation and lateral luxation. In: Andreasen JO, Andreasen FM, Andersson L, editors. Textbook and color atlas of traumatic injuries to the teeth. 5th ed. Hoboken: Wiley-Blackwell; 2019. p. 450–68.
11. Nikoui M, Kenny DJ, Barrett EJ. Clinical outcomes for permanent incisor luxations in a pediatric population. III. Lateral luxations. Dent Traumatol. 2003;19:280–5.
12. Lauridsen E, Hermann N, Gerds TA, Ahrensburg SS, Kreiborg S, Andreasen JO. Dental trauma. Combination injuries 3. The risk of pulp necrosis in permanent teeth with extrusion or lateral luxation injuries and concomitant crown fractures without pulp exposure. Dent Traumatol. 2012;28:379–85.
13. Andreasen FM. Transient apical breakdown and its relation to color and sensibility changes. Endod Dent Traumatol. 1986;2:9–19.
14. Cohenca N, Karni S, Rotstein I. Transient apical breakdown following tooth luxation. Dent Traumatol. 2003;19:289–91.
15. Skaare AB, Jacobsen I. Dental injuries in Norwegians aged 7-18 years. Dent Traumatol. 2003;19:67–71.
16. Ziegler AM. Analysis of a comprehensive dental trauma database: an epidemiologic study of traumatic dental injuries to the permanent dentition. Dissertation, The Ohio State University; 2014.
17. Hermann NV, Lauridsen E, Ahrensburg SS, Gerds TA, Andreasen JO. Periodontal healing complications following extrusive and lateral luxation in the permanent dentiton. A longitudinal cohort study. Dent Traumatol. 2012;28:394–402.

18. Andreasen JO, Andreasen FM, Tsilingaridis G. Intrusive luxation. In: Andreasen JO, Andreasen FM, Andersson L, editors. Textbook and color atlas of traumatic injuries to the teeth. 5th ed. Hoboken: Wiley-Blackwell; 2019. p. 469–85.
19. Andreasen JO, Bakland LK, Matras RC, Andreasen FM. Traumatic intrusion of permanent teeth. Part 1. An epidemiological study of 216 intruded permanent teeth. Dent Traumatol. 2006;22:83–9.
20. Tsilingaridis G, Malmgren B, Andreasen JO, Malmgren O. Intrusive luxation of 60 permanent incisors: a retrospective study of treatment and outcome. Dent Traumatol. 2012;28:416–22.
21. Tsilingaridis G, Malmgren B, Andreasen JO, Wigen TI, Maseng Aas AL, Malmgren O. Scandinavian multi-center study on the treatment of 168 patients with 230 intruded permanent teeth – a retrospective cohort study. Dent Traumatol. 2016;32:353–60.

Permanent Tooth Avulsion Injuries

Tooth avulsion results in the complete displacement of the tooth out of the socket. Frequently, the tooth is brought in to the clinic in a jar of milk or a plastic bag. Occasionally, the tooth is not found at the site of injury. The clinical findings of an empty tooth socket along with a radiograph confirming that the tooth was not intruded or fractured confirm the diagnosis (Fig. 8.1). There are likely additional hard and soft tissue injuries that accompany an avulsion.

Avulsion of one or more teeth is a relatively uncommon injury. Published studies report a frequency of between 0.5 and 16% of traumatic dental injuries to permanent teeth [1]. The majority are the result of sports injuries and fights. In a U.S. study of traumatic dental injuries treated at a Children's Hospital, of 1218 teeth with traumatic dental injuries, 6% were avulsions of permanent teeth. The most common age for this injury was between 11 and 15 years [2]. Other studies report that avulsions are more likely to occur in children between 7 and 9 years of age, when the permanent incisors are erupting [1, 3]. In a 12-year retrospective study based in Brazil, Mesquita et al. found that the most common age for avulsed permanent teeth was between 6 and 10 years of age and the most common etiology was bicycle accidents [4].

Avulsion of a permanent tooth results in injury to the pulp and periodontium. The survival of periodontal ligament cells depends on the proper handling of the tooth and either immediate replantation or storage in appropriate storage media. Minimizing extraoral dry time is critical to the survival of these periodontal ligament cells as well.

R. L. Slayton, E. A. Palmer, *Traumatic Dental Injuries in Children*,
https://doi.org/10.1007/978-3-030-25793-4_8

Fig. 8.1 Avulsion of permanent maxillary right central incisor (**a**). Radiograph confirms that the tooth was not intruded and that there were no concomitant dental injuries (**b**)

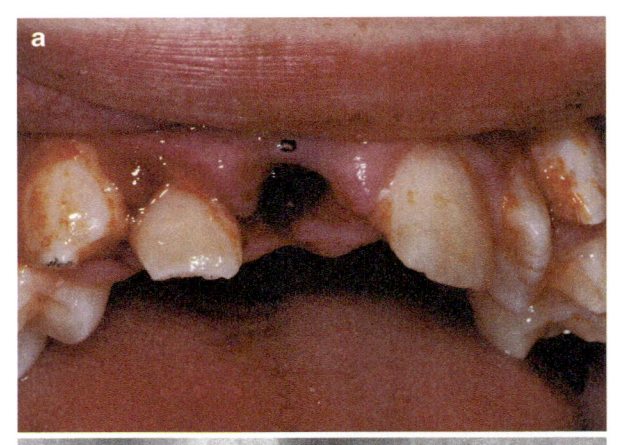

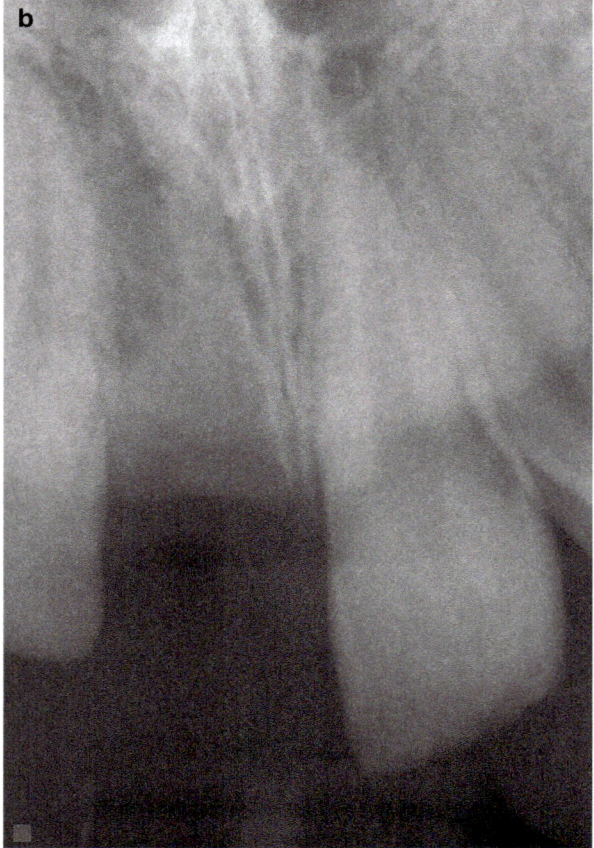

8.1   Pulpal Reactions

Reactions of the pulp tissue following tooth avulsion have been studied in a number of animal models including cats, dogs, and monkeys [1, 5]. In one of the early studies, Anderson et al, classified the pulp and dentin responses after extraction and immediate replantation demonstrating a range of responses including reparative dentin, internal resorption, and pulp necrosis [5]. Studies in humans are more challenging and have primarily used premolars that were planned for extraction for orthodontic purposes. In one study by Fiane et al., 57 premolars were extracted, immediately replanted, and then evaluated histologically at 1, 2, 3, 6, 12, and 24 weeks [6]. There was a mix of immature and mature teeth in the study sample. Radiographs were taken before the first extraction and at the time of the second extraction. The authors found that regeneration of vasculature in immature teeth occurred between 3 and 6 weeks with evidence of tertiary dentin being formed. This was less frequently seen in mature teeth [6]. This study may be more relevant for teeth that are autotransplanted than for traumatically avulsed teeth, because in autotransplantation, the tooth is immediately replanted whereas in a traumatic avulsion, there is often a delay in replantation.

Pulpal healing is more likely in teeth with open apices, and the guidelines recommend promoting revascularization of the pulp and avoidance of pulp infection when immature teeth are avulsed [7]. Mature teeth with closed apices are very likely to become necrotic following avulsion and replantation, so endodontic treatment is part of the treatment guideline for these teeth [7].

8.2   Periodontal Reactions

The other healing complication associated with permanent tooth avulsion is related to the periodontal ligament cells. At the time of the avulsion, viable periodontal ligament cells remain on the root surface. If these cells are allowed to dry out, they become non-viable. If hydration is maintained with a medium that does not cause damage to the cells, they will remain viable for a limited time and can repair following replantation. As the healing process continues, and inflammation decreases, replacement cementum is formed [8]. When periodontal ligament cells are allowed to dry out, they trigger a severe inflammatory response over the entire root surface resulting in attachment of bone to the root surface rather than replacement cementum [8]. This process of ankylosis has negative consequences in the growing child because vertical growth of the alveolar process is inhibited resulting in the infraposition of the ankylosed tooth or teeth [9]. This creates an esthetic issue when teeth are located in the anterior region and is a challenge to treat, since the affected teeth cannot be repositioned orthodontically. Treatment options for ankylosed teeth will be discussed in more detail in Chap. 9. Over time, replacement resorption will cause the root to be resorbed and bone to take its place. This process may take 4–5 years in adolescents and young adults and is a much longer process in older adults [9].

Andreasen et al. described four different periodontal ligament healing patterns, based on histologic studies of replanted teeth in humans and animals. The first is the regeneration of a normal periodontal ligament that is evident histologically in about 4 weeks. The radiographic appearance is normal with no signs of root resorption and clinically, the tooth is in its normal position with normal mobility and percussion tone [1]. The second pattern demonstrates repair-related resorption. In this case, there are histologic signs of surface resorption which is self-limiting. This surface resorption may not be seen radiographically. Clinically the tooth is in the normal position with normal percussion sounds and the pulp is usually vital [1]. The third pattern includes ankylosis-related resorption. The histologic findings show a fusion between the alveolar bone and the root surface that may occur as early as 2 weeks after replantation. Ankylosis may be progressive or transient, but when the periodontal ligament cells are removed prior to replantation, the pattern is progressive. In the early stages, ankylosis may not be visible radiographically, but later (6 months or more), there is a loss of the periodontal ligament space and eventual replacement of root with bone. Clinically, the tooth does not demonstrate physiologic mobility and in a growing patient, will appear to be in infraocclusion. The percussion tone is distinctive and is described as being a high tone when compared to the adjacent non-ankylosed tooth [1]. Infection-related resorption is the fourth pattern of healing described by Andreasen et al. [1]. In this situation, inflammatory resorption is evident histologically in the periodontal tissue and bone. It is often a very rapid process, particularly in younger patients. Radiographically, signs of infection-related resorption may be seen as early as 2 weeks after replantation and appear as semicircular cavitations on the root surface and adjacent bone. The clinical findings include mobility and extrusion of the tooth as well as sensitivity to percussion [1]. These healing patterns make it clear how important it is to maintain the vitality of the periodontal ligament cells by either immediate replantation or placement in a suitable transport medium.

8.3   Treatment Guidelines

Evidence to support treatment guidelines are limited to experimental and clinical studies. It is very difficult to perform a randomized clinical trial with sufficient numbers of subjects. Trauma centers in Denmark, Sweden, and other countries have been able to compile outcomes from individuals with traumatic dental injuries, in some cases over a 20–30 year follow-up time frame. This provides a unique and rich source of data to assess both successes and failures of treatment approaches. The current guidelines for treatment of permanent tooth avulsions were initially published in 2001 and are updated on a regular basis with the most current version published in 2012 [7].

As will be described below and demonstrated in the decision trees in Figs. 8.2 and 8.3, the treatment guidelines vary based on the maturity of the avulsed tooth, the time the tooth has been out of the socket and whether it has been stored dry or in an appropriate transport medium. All of these factors affect the treatment decisions and the prognosis of the tooth.

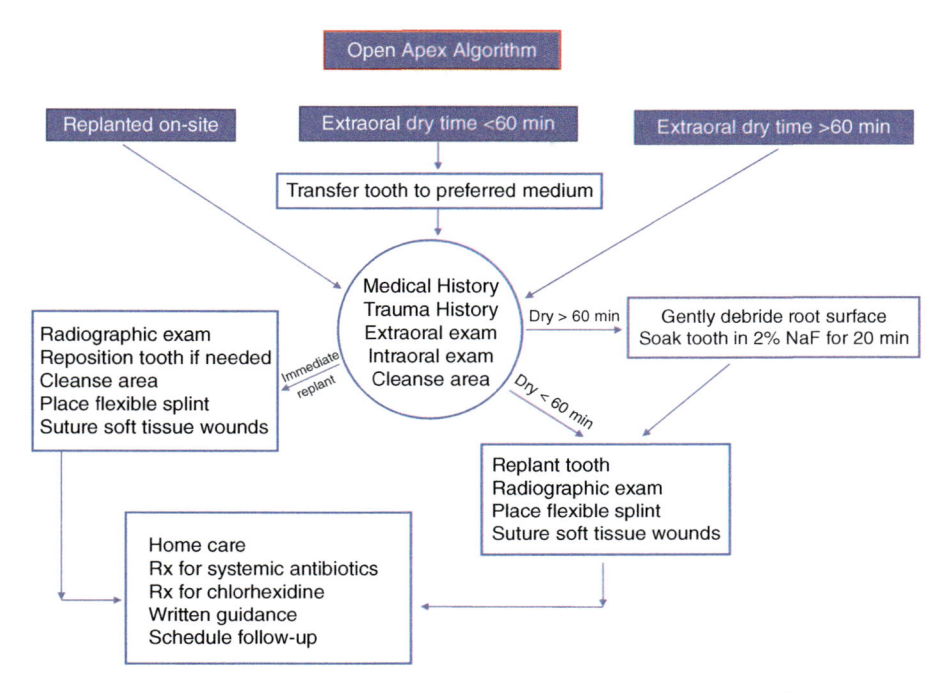

Fig. 8.2 Algorithm for treatment of avulsed immature (open apex) permanent teeth

8.4 Triage Protocol

Frequently, the first communication with a caregiver regarding a child's traumatic dental injury is over the phone. It is essential that the front desk staff members know the right questions to ask and are able to provide guidance to the caregiver about what steps they should follow before arriving at the office. A trauma script is recommended so that important facts are not forgotten. An example of a script is shown below. When the injury involves avulsion of a tooth, it is important to know right away if this is a primary or permanent tooth, so the age of the child should be one of the first questions asked. The next priority should be to determine if the child's injury is severe enough that they should go to the emergency department first rather than the dental office. This may be difficult to determine over the phone, but questions that identify the extent of the injury will be a useful guide. If it is determined that this is most likely a permanent tooth, the caregiver should be instructed to either replant it in the socket or place it in cold milk and bring the child immediately to the office. If there is debris on the tooth, it can be rinsed briefly under cold water before replanting.

Triage script for front desk or after-hours call service
How old is your child?
Did the child lose consciousness?
If a tooth was knocked out, was it found?
When did the accident happen?
How did the accident happen?
Who witnessed the accident?
Where did the accident happen?

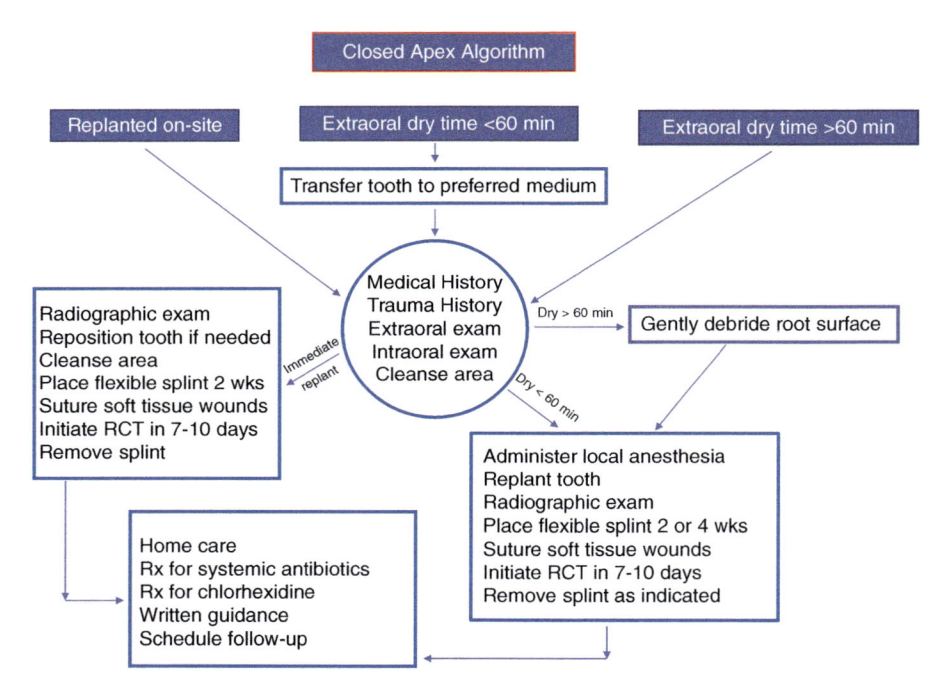

Fig. 8.3 Algorithm for treatment of avulsed mature (closed apex) permanent teeth

If the injury occurs after-hours, the caregiver may either decide to go directly to the emergency department or to call the dentist's after-hours number. Dentists are expected to be available after-hours to manage dental emergencies for their patients of record. If they are not available, arrangements should be made to have a colleague cover emergencies when needed. Delay in treating an avulsed permanent tooth significantly compromises its prognosis. As mentioned previously, many small community hospitals do not have a dentist on staff. If the patient presents to the emergency department and there is no dentist on staff, it is incumbent on the medical team to have the knowledge and ability to replant the avulsed tooth prior to referring the patient to a local dentist. One study of emergency room physician knowledge of dental trauma management showed that although 61% of respondents were somewhat confident in managing dental trauma, 41% were comfortable, and 19% were not comfortable replanting an avulsed tooth [10]. In another study, a survey of both emergency room nurses and physicians, showed that there was a lack of knowledge in both groups about the proper management of avulsed teeth [11]. Since emergency room physicians and nurses are often the first point of contact for traumatic dental injuries, this is concerning and suggests an opportunity for additional training for emergency room staff members.

Another scenario that must be considered is the child who does not have an established dental home and/or has limited access to care. When children in this group have urgent dental needs, especially after-hours, the hospital emergency room may be their only option. If they live far from a regional hospital, this will cause additional delay in receiving urgent needed treatment.

8.5 Transport/Storage Media

Maintaining the viability of periodontal ligament cells is the first priority related to the prognosis of the tooth. If the tooth cannot be replanted immediately, for whatever reason, it should be placed in a suitable transport/storage medium. Over the years, a number of studies have been done to determine the best medium to keep cells alive for the longest period of time. Udoye et al. recently reviewed all the transport media that have been studied and concluded that the most practical choice because of its general availability, is cold milk [12]. These authors provided very useful information about the features of 15 different media. The characteristics of these agents are summarized in Table 8.1. More recently, Osmanovic et al. performed a systematic review of storage media and its effect on periodontal ligament cell viability [13]. Their recommendation was in agreement with Udoye et al. due to

Table 8.1 Summary of transport media

	pH	Enhanced cell viability	Maximum storage period
Reasonably available			
Hank's Balanced Salt Solution	7.4	Yes	24 h
Milk	6.5–7.2	Yes	2–3 h
Normal saline	7.4	Somewhat	1 h
Saliva	–	Yes	30 min
Water	7.4	No	Rinse only
Gatorade	2.92	No	–
Contact lens solution	–	No	–
Coconut water	4.1	No	–
Not easily available			
ViaSpan	7.4	Yes	>24 h
Eagle's medium	6.8?	Yes	
Dubelco's medium	6.87	Yes	
Propolis	8.5	Yes	6 h
Egg white	8.6–9.38	Yes	24 h

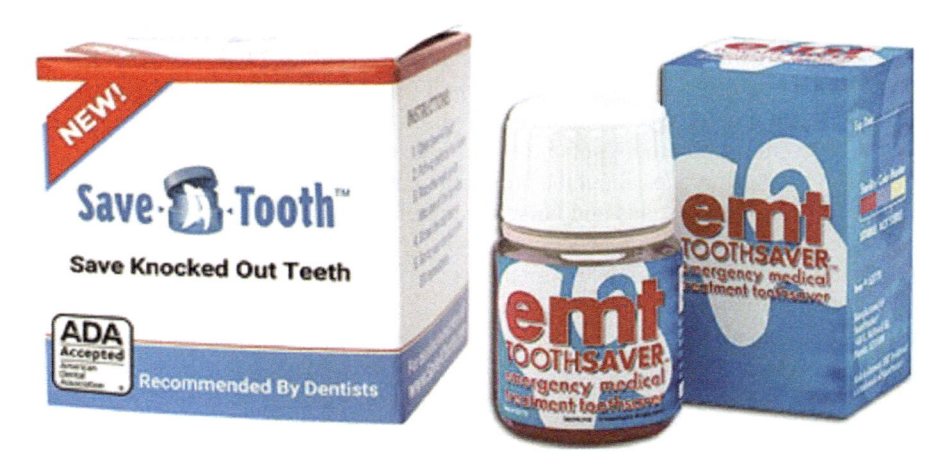

Fig. 8.4 Examples of tooth preservation kits available online

the general availability and low cost of milk. However, it should be noted that cell viability is only maintained for a relatively short period (2 h) when the tooth is stored in milk. If there will be a delay in replanting the tooth, it should be transferred as soon as possible to a medium such as Hank's Balanced Salt Solution (HBSS) which has a maximum storage period of 24 h [12]. This solution is available in a tooth saving kit from pharmacies or online for less than $20 (Fig. 8.4). It has a 2-year shelf life at room temperature and should be a standard part of any emergency kit at homes, schools, hospitals, physician, and dental offices.

8.6 Immature Teeth Replanted Immediately or Within 60 min

Teeth with open root apices (greater than 1 mm) are considered to be immature and are treated differently because of their increased ability for revascularization. The other factors related to patients with open apex teeth are that the child is young, may be anxious, and uncooperative for the needed treatment. Also, in very young teeth, the root is only partially formed, so root canal treatment is challenging. Revascularization will allow continued root development and should be the primary consideration for pulp management.

8.6.1 Treatment Recommendations

Treatment is dictated by the time the tooth is out of the socket and whether or not it was stored in appropriate transport medium and the degree of root development. The ideal treatment is for the tooth to be replanted at the scene of the injury within 15 min. The PDL cells have a high probability of surviving in this situation. When

Table 8.2 Splint duration based on root apex development and time out of socket or transport medium

Description of injury/time out of socket	Splint duration (weeks)
Open apex < 60 min	2
Open apex > 60 min	4
Closed apex < 60 min	2
Closed apex > 60 min	4

this is not possible, the next best option is for the tooth to be placed in an acceptable transport medium such as HBSS or cold milk. Do not place the tooth in water. If the tooth is placed in HBSS or milk within 60 min, the PDL cells may be viable. Emergency rooms, sport teams, and schools are encouraged to have emergency tooth kits on hand, but data has demonstrated that this is more the exception than the rule. When the avulsed tooth is dry for greater than 60 min, the PDL cells are most likely not viable. The various treatment scenarios are described below.

In this treatment scenario, the tooth was either replanted on site or was placed in appropriate transport medium in a timely way. In either case, it is important to confirm the time of avulsion and length of time the tooth was out of the mouth before being replanted or placed in transport medium.

If the tooth was replanted on site, verify the position of the tooth clinically and radiographically. If not yet replanted, administer local anesthesia, remove any debris on the root, and replant the tooth. If there has been a delay in seeking treatment, the coagulum in the socket may make it difficult to reposition the tooth to its original position. In this case, the socket may need to be gently curetted first. If there are any soft tissue lacerations, they should be managed after replanting the tooth and placing the splint.

Place a flexible splint for 2 weeks (Table 8.2). Research has shown that it is important to provide support but also to allow healing of the periodontal ligament and gingival fibers. Rigid splints are no longer recommended, as they increase the risk for root resorption [7].

Verify up to date tetanus immunization. If not up to date, send patient to their primary care provider for a booster.

Prescribe systemic antibiotics—Doxycycline is recommended if the child is over 12 years, Pen VK if under 12 years due to the risk of tetracycline staining in developing teeth.

Systemic antibiotic prescriptions based on age and allergy to penicillin
- If *over* 12 years of age and *less than* 45 kg:
  Doxycycline 4.4 mg/kg/day q 12h on day 1, then 2.2 mg/kg/day q12h for 7 days
- If *over* 12 years of age and *greater than* 45 kg:
  Doxycycline 200 mg q 12h on day 1, then 100 mg q12h for 7 days
- If *under* 12 years of age and *less than* 45 kg:
  Pen VK 50 mg/kg/day divided q 6–8h for 7 days
- If *under* 12 years of age and *greater than* 45 kg:

> Pen VK 500 mg PO q 6h for 7 days
> - If *under* 12 years of age, *less than* 45 kg and *Penicillin allergic*: Clindamycin 10–25 mg/kg/day PO divided q6–8h for 7 days
> - If *under* 12 years of age, *greater than* 45 kg and *Penicillin allergic*: Clindamycin 250 mg PO q 6h for 7 days

Prescribe chlorhexidine rinse with detailed, age specific instructions for use.

> Chlorhexidine 0.12% oral rinse
> Rinse gently twice daily with 5 mL for 30 s and then expectorate.
> NPO 30 min.
> If unable to rinse, apply to teeth and gums twice daily using a soft toothbrush and then expectorate excess. Do not rinse with water for 30 min.

Provide family with detailed, written postoperative instructions for home care including the timing of follow-up visits.

> **Patient Instructions**
> Restrict diet to soft food for up to 2 weeks.
> Avoid participation in sports.
> Maintain good oral hygiene to improve healing of oral tissues.
> Brush with a soft toothbrush and rinse with chlorhexidine 0.12% twice daily.
> For young children, it is recommended to use chlorhexidine without alcohol (Paroex® Sunstar GUM; Perioguard alcohol free—Colgate Oral Pharmaceuticals).

It is important that caregivers understand the potential sequelae related to avulsion injuries including signs and symptoms to be aware of. At the time of the injury, even if these outcomes are clearly explained, they may not be remembered due to the emotions surrounding the traumatic injury of their child. For this reason, it is recommended that this information be provided in written form so that it can be referred to at a later date.

> **Potential sequelae following avulsion**
> Inflammation of tissues surrounding the root, causing resorption
> Fusion of the tooth root to the bone (ankylosis)
> Infection of the tooth or supporting tissues
> Swelling of the gums as a sign of infection
> Tooth loss due to infection or root resorption
> Tooth discoloration (yellow or gray)
> Tooth submergence resulting in the tooth being shorter than the adjacent tooth

8.6.2 Follow-Up

After 2 weeks, the patient should be seen for clinical and radiographic examination and removal of the splint. Additional clinical and radiographic examination should be done at 4 weeks, 3 months, 6 months, and annually for 5 years [7]. At each visit, the root apex is monitored for continued root development and possible pulpal obliteration.

8.6.3 Prognosis

The most common sequelae are pulp necrosis, pulpal obliteration, ankylosis, and inflammatory root resorption [14] (Fig. 8.5). For immature teeth, it is recommended

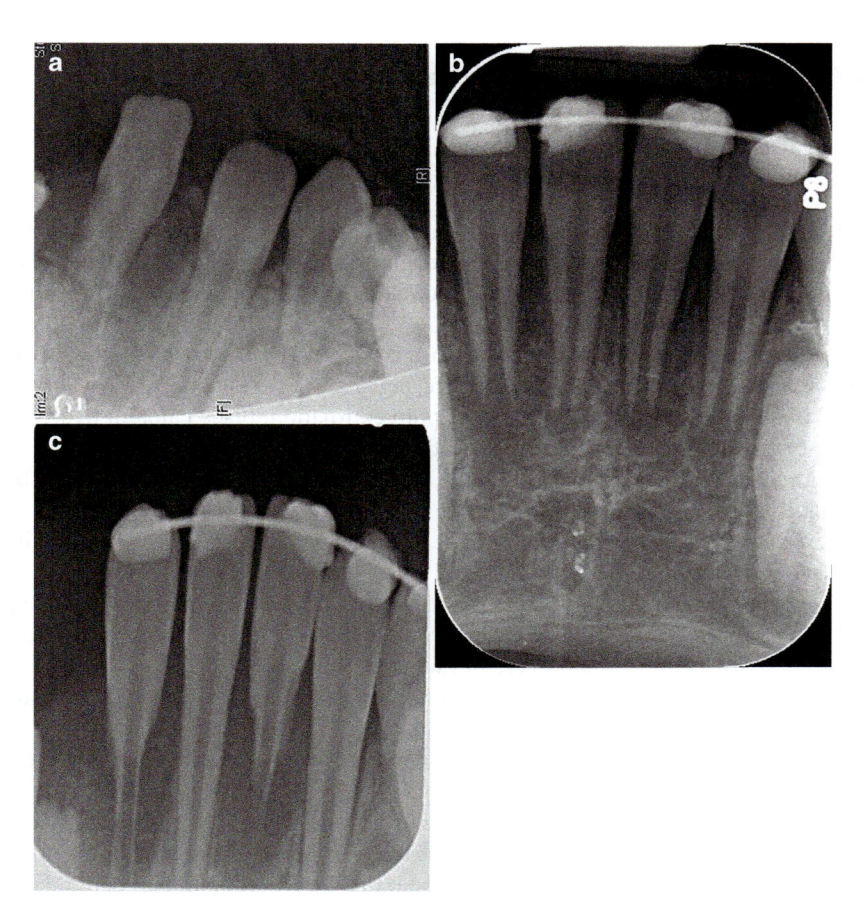

Fig. 8.5 Avulsed permanent mandibular central and lateral incisors (**a**). Stored in milk less than 60 min; replanted and splinted following guidelines (**b**). Due to patient anxiety, RCT not completed within 7–10 days. Returned on day 45 (**c**) and required extraction of lower left central incisor and lower right lateral incisor and root canal treatment of the lower left lateral incisor and lower right central incisor in the operating room under general anesthesia

to delay root canal treatment to allow pulp regeneration. If this doesn't occur or if there is evidence of pulp necrosis, root canal treatment should be initiated.

Souza et al. performed a meta-analysis to evaluate the incidence of different types of root resorption following replantation of avulsed permanent teeth [15]. The included studies reported on both immature and mature teeth. Replacement root resorption (ankylosis) was the most frequently reported type of root resorption with an incidence of 51%. The incidence of inflammatory root resorption was 23.2% and surface root resorption was 13.3%. The least common type of resorption was internal root resorption, with an incidence of 1.2%. There was no significant difference between teeth with open or closed apices. These findings are similar to previously published results. For this meta-analysis, the overall evidence was considered very low, mainly due to risk of bias and the observational study design that is common in studies of traumatic dental injuries.

8.7 Immature Teeth with Extraoral Dry Time Greater Than 60 min

8.7.1 Treatment Recommendations

When avulsed teeth have extraoral dry time greater than 60 min, the PDL cells will not survive and should be removed by cleaning the root surface with gauze. Then, the tooth is placed in 2% sodium fluoride solution for 20 min to minimize root resorption after replantation [7].

If possible, a pulpectomy may be performed in hand prior to replantation. This is particularly relevant for children who are perceived to be uncooperative for root canal treatment in the near future. After pulp extirpation, place calcium hydroxide in the canal space to encourage apexification.

Administer local anesthetic, irrigate the socket with sterile saline, and then replant tooth.

Verify position of the tooth clinically and radiographically and place a flexible splint for 4 weeks (Table 8.2).

Prescribe systemic antibiotics as described previously, based on the child's age and history of allergy to penicillin. Confirm that tetanus immunization is up to date and refer to the child's primary care physician if needed.

Prescribe chlorhexidine rinse with clear instructions for use. This is the same protocol as for teeth replanted within 60 min.

Provide family with detailed, written postoperative instructions for home care including the timing of follow-up visits.

It is important that caregivers understand the potential sequelae related to avulsion injuries including signs and symptoms to be aware of. At the time of the injury, even if these outcomes are clearly explained, they may not be remembered due to the emotions surrounding the traumatic injury of their child. For this reason, it is recommended that this information be provided in written form so that it can be referred to at a later date. This information is the same as that provided for immature teeth that are replanted within 60 min.

Replantation of an avulsed permanent tooth may not be appropriate for children with severe cardiac disease, severe seizure disorder, immunocompromised status, or severe developmental delay. The dentist must weigh the risks and benefits and provide thorough informed consent to the family regarding the prognosis and risk for infection.

8.7.2 Follow-Up

The child should be seen for clinical and radiographic evaluation at 2–4 weeks, 3 months, 6 months, annually for 5 years [7]. The splint is removed at the 4-week evaluation.

8.7.3 Prognosis

The most common sequelae are pulp necrosis, pulpal obliteration, ankylosis, and inflammatory root resorption [14] (Fig. 8.5a–c). For immature teeth with extraoral dry time greater than 60 min, pulp regeneration is unlikely and pulp extirpation should be done within 7–10 days followed by apexification with calcium hydroxide.

8.8 Mature Teeth Replanted Immediately or Within 60 min

The primary difference with avulsion of mature teeth is that pulp regeneration is unlikely. Therefore, root canal treatment is required and should be completed within 7–10 days of replantation. As with immature teeth, the clinical scenarios and treatment decisions are related to the extraoral dry time and type of transport media.

8.8.1 Treatment Recommendations

In this treatment scenario, the tooth was either replanted on site or was placed in appropriate transport medium in a timely way. In either case, it is important to confirm the time of avulsion and time the tooth was out of the mouth before being replanted or placed in transport medium. Document the type of transport medium and length of time the tooth was in that medium.

Fig. 8.6 Replantation of avulsed maxillary central incisor and verification of position with radiograph (**a**). Flexible splint in place (**b**)

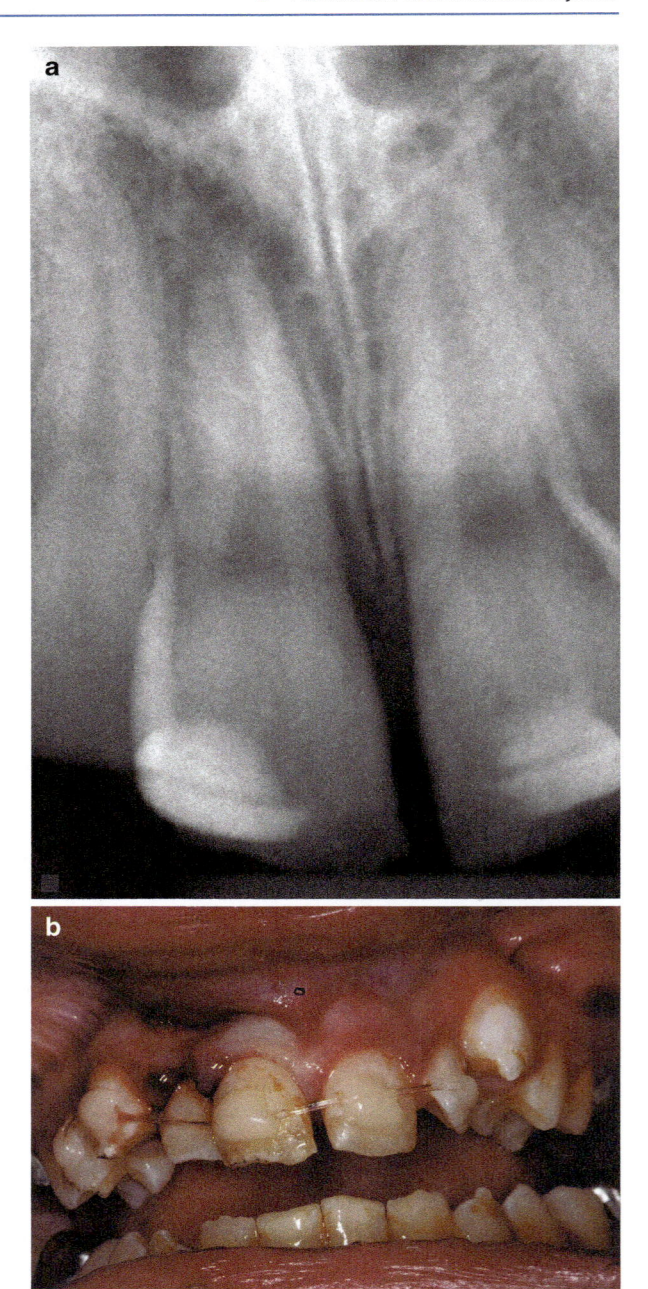

If the tooth was replanted on site, verify the position of the tooth clinically and radiographically (Fig. 8.6a, b). If not yet replanted, administer local anesthesia, rinse off any debris on the root surface, and replant the tooth. If there has been a delay in seeking treatment, the coagulum in the socket may make it difficult to reposition the tooth to its original position. In this case, the socket may need to be gently curetted first. If there are any soft tissue lacerations, they should be managed after replanting the tooth and placing the splint.

Place a flexible splint for 2 weeks (Table 8.2). Research has shown that it is important to provide support but also to allow healing of the periodontal ligament and gingival fibers. Rigid splints are no longer recommended, as they increase the risk for root resorption [7].

Suture any soft tissue lacerations.

Verify up to date tetanus immunization. If not up to date, send patient to their primary care provider for a booster.

Prescribe systemic antibiotics as described previously, based on the child's age and history of allergy to penicillin.

Prescribe chlorhexidine rinse with clear instructions for use. This is the same protocol as for teeth replanted within 60 min.

Provide the family with detailed, written postoperative instructions for home care including the timing of follow-up visits.

It is important that caregivers understand the potential sequelae related to avulsion injuries including signs and symptoms to be aware of. At the time of the injury, even if these outcomes are clearly explained, they may not be remembered due to the emotions surrounding the traumatic injury of their child. For this reason, it is recommended that this information be provided in written form so that it can be referred to at a later date. This information is the same as that provided for immature teeth that are replanted within 60 min.

Root canal treatment should be initiated within 7–10 days (prior to splint removal). Consider pulp extirpation at time of replantation or root canal treatment in hand, especially for children where cooperation could be an issue.

8.8.2 Follow-Up

If root canal treatment was not done at the time of replantation, it should be completed in 7–10 days (Fig. 8.7a). Often this is done before removing the splint. The splint is removed at 2 weeks (Fig. 8.7b). Clinical and radiographic examination is done at 4 weeks, 3 months, 6 months, and annually for 5 years [7]. At each visit, evaluate for signs of infraposition, inflammation, and ankylosis. Consider decoronation when infraposition is >1 mm. This will be described in more detail in Chap. 9.

Fig. 8.7 Root canal treatment was completed prior to splint removal and within 7–10 days of the injury (**a**). At 2-week follow-up visit, the splint is removed (**b**)

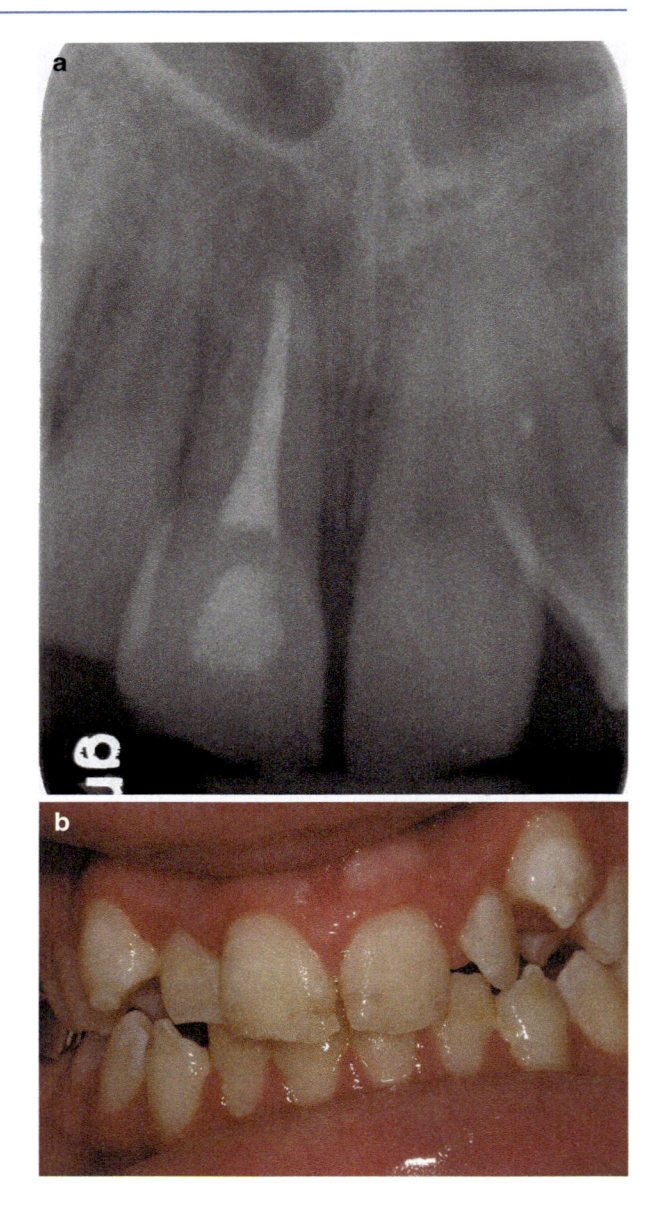

Replantation may not be appropriate for children with severe cardiac disease, severe seizure disorder, immunocompromised status, or severe developmental delay. The dentist must weigh the risks and benefits and provide thorough informed consent to the family regarding the prognosis and risk for infection.

8.8.3 Prognosis

The most common sequelae are pulp necrosis, pulpal obliteration, ankylosis, and inflammatory root resorption [14]. For mature teeth regardless of the extraoral dry time, pulp regeneration is unlikely and root canal treatment should be completed within 7–10 days.

Souza et al. performed a meta-analysis to evaluate the incidence of different types of root resorption following replantation of avulsed permanent teeth [15]. The included studies reported on both immature and mature teeth. Replacement root resorption (ankylosis) was the most frequently reported type of root resorption with an incidence of 51%. The incidence of inflammatory root resorption was 23.2% and surface root resorption was 13.3%. The least common type of resorption was internal root resorption with an incidence of 1.2%. There was no significant difference between teeth with open or closed apices. These findings are similar to previously published results. For this meta-analysis, the overall evidence was considered very low, mainly due to risk of bias and the observational study design that is common in studies of traumatic dental injuries.

8.9 Mature Teeth with Extraoral Dry Time Greater Than 60 min

When mature avulsed teeth have extraoral dry time greater than 60 min, the PDL cells will not survive and should be removed by cleaning the root surface with gauze. Place the tooth in 2% sodium fluoride solution for 20 min to minimize root resorption after replantation [7].

8.9.1 Treatment Recommendations

If possible, perform a pulpectomy or root canal treatment in hand prior to replantation. This is particularly relevant for children who are perceived to be uncooperative for root canal treatment in the near future. After pulp extirpation, place calcium hydroxide in the canal space and plan on completing the root canal treatment within 7–10 days.

Administer local anesthetic, irrigate the socket with sterile saline, and then replant tooth.

Verify position of tooth clinically and radiographically and place a flexible splint for 4 weeks (Table 8.2).

Suture any soft tissue lacerations.

Verify up to date tetanus immunization. If not up to date, send patient to their primary care provider for a booster.

Prescribe systemic antibiotics as described previously, based on the child's age and history of allergy to penicillin.

Prescribe chlorhexidine rinse with clear instructions for use. This is the same protocol as for teeth replanted within 60 min.

Provide the family with detailed, written postoperative instructions for home care including the timing of follow-up visits.

8.9.2 Follow-Up

Clinical and radiographic evaluation at 2–4 weeks, 3 months, 6 months, and annually for 5 years. The splint is removed after 4 weeks. Most common sequelae are ankylosis, inflammatory root resorption, and tooth loss. Evaluate for signs of infraposition, infection, and inflammation. Consider decoronation when infraposition >1 mm. This will be described in more detail in Chap. 9.

In cases of tooth loss due to severe inflammatory root resorption, autotransplantation may be considered. This is described in detail in Andreasen et al. [16] and briefly discussed in Chap. 9 of this text.

8.9.3 Prognosis

It is important that caregivers understand the potential sequelae related to avulsion injuries including signs and symptoms to be aware of. At the time of the injury, even if these outcomes are clearly explained, they may not be remembered due to the emotions surrounding the traumatic injury of their child. For this reason, it is recommended that this information be provided in written form so that it can be referred to at a later date. This information is the same as that provided for immature teeth that are replanted within 60 min.

Replantation may not be appropriate for children with severe cardiac disease, severe seizure disorder, immunocompromised status, or severe developmental delay. The dentist must weigh the risks and benefits and provide thorough informed consent to the family regarding the prognosis and risk for infection.

References

1. Andreasen JO, Andreasen FM, Tsilingaridis G. Avulsions. In: Andreasen JO, Andreasen FM, Andersson L, editors. Textbook and color atlas of traumatic injuries to the teeth. 5th ed. Hoboken: Wiley-Blackwell; 2019. p. 486–528.
2. Ziegler AM. Analysis of a comprehensive dental trauma database: an epidemiologic study of traumatic dental injuries to the permanent dentition. Dissertation, The Ohio State University; 2014.
3. Andreasen JO, Borum M, Jacobsen HL, Andreasen FM. Replantation of 400 traumatically avulsed permanent incisors. I. Diagnosis of healing complications. Endod Dent Traumatol. 1995;11:51–8.
4. Mesquita BC, Soares PBF, Moura CCG, Roscoe MG, Paiva SM, Soares CJ. A 12-year retrospective study of avulsion cases in a public Brazilian Dental Trauma Service. Braz Dent J. 2017;28:749–56.

5. Anderson AW, Sharav Y, Massler M. Reparative dentine formation and pulp morphology. Oral Surg Oral Med Oral Pathol. 1968;26:837–47.
6. Fiane JE, Breivik M, Vandevska-Radunovic V. A histomorphometric and radiographic study of replanted human premolars. Eur J Orthod. 2014;36:641–8.
7. Andersson L, Andreasen JO, Day P, Heithersay G, Trope M, DiAngelis AJ, Kenny DJ, Sigurdsson A, Bourguignon C, Flores MT, Hicks ML, Lenzi AR, Malmgren B, Moule AJ, Tsukiboshi M. Guidelines for the management of traumatic dental injuries: 2. Avulsion of permanent teeth. Dent Traumatol. 2012;28:88–96.
8. Trope M, Barnett F, Sigurdsson A, Chivian N. The role of endodontics after dental traumatic injuries. In: Hargreaves KM, Berman LH, editors. Cohen's pathways of the pulp. 11th ed. St. Louis: Elsevier; 2016. p. 758–92.
9. Malmgren B, Malmgren O, Andersson L. Dentoalveolar ankylosis, decoronation and alveolar bone preservation. In: Andreasen JO, Andreasen FM, Andersson L, editors. Textbook and color atlas of traumatic injuries to the teeth. 5th ed. Hoboken: Wiley-Blackwell; 2019. p. 834–52.
10. Cully M, Cully J, Nietrt PJ, Titus MO. Physician confidence in dental trauma treatment and the introduction of a dental trauma decision-making pathway for the Pediatric Emergency Department. Pediatr Emerg Care. 2018; https://doi.org/10.1097/PEC.0000000000001479. [Epub ahead of print].
11. Iyer SS, Panigrahi A, Sharma S. Knowledge and awareness of first aid of avulsed tooth among physicians and nurses of Hospital Emergency Department. J Pharm Bioallied Sci. 2017;9:94–8.
12. Udoye CI, Jafarzadeh H, Abbott PV. Transport media for avulsed teeth: a review. Aust Endod J. 2012;38:129–36.
13. Osmanovic A, Halilovic S, Kurtovic-Kozaric A, Hadziabdic N. Evaluation of periodontal ligament cell viability in different storage media based on human PDL cell culture experiments-A systematic review. Dent Traumatol. 2018;34:384–93.
14. Andreasen JO, editor. The dental trauma guide. San Diego: International Association of Dental Traumatology; 2012.
15. Souza BDM, Dutra KL, Kuntze MM, Bortoluzzi EA, Flores-Mir C, Reyes-Carmona J, Felippe WT, Porporatti AL, De Luca Canto G. Incidence of root resorption after the replantation of avulsed teeth: a meta-analysis. J Endod. 2018;44:1216–27.
16. Andreasen JO, Andersson L, Tsukiboshi M, Czochrowska EM. Autotransplantation of teeth to the anterior region. In: Andreasen JO, Andreasen FM, Andersson L, editors. Textbook and color atlas of traumatic injuries to the teeth. 5th ed. Hoboken: Wiley-Blackwell; 2019. p. 853–77.

Sequelae and Management Options

9

Unfortunately, the effects of a traumatic injury to the oral cavity may continue long past the initial evaluation and treatment. Thus, it is very important that the child that has experienced a traumatic dental injury be followed and reevaluated at the appropriate time intervals recommended for the particular injury. Both clinical and radiographic examinations may be necessary as many of the sequelae are present in the pulp chamber, the roots, and succedaneous tooth buds. Even still, it is impossible to know what is happening at the histopathological level, but some sequelae are more often associated with specific traumatic dental injuries.

9.1 Tooth Discoloration

Immediately following an injury, the pulp will become hyperemic due to increased blood flow to the injured tooth. The coronal portion of a tooth with pulpal hyperemia may appear to have a pinkish/reddish tint clinically and exhibit symptoms of reversible pulpitis. Whether or not these symptoms are transient is dependent on the extent of the injury to the neurovascular bundle and periodontal ligament (PDL), as well as the size of the apical foramen and the presence/absence of bacteria in the healing area [1–3].

If the hyperemia and inflammation ruptures the capillaries within the traumatized tooth, the pigments from the extra blood may discolor the tooth a reddish, yellow, or gray color. This discoloration will be evident in the first couple of weeks following the injury. This color change may be transient if the blood is reabsorbed or indefinite if the blood spreads into the dentin tubules. A discolored tooth due to internal hemorrhage may retain its vitality; however, if the discoloration appears months or years following an injury, that tooth likely has developed a necrotic pulp [2, 3] (Fig. 9.1).

Multiple studies have shown that when primary teeth are discolored, they are more likely to be necrotic or partially necrotic [4–6]. It is important to evaluate the tooth for other symptoms of pulp necrosis such as abscess, fistula, periapical lesion,

© Springer Nature Switzerland AG 2020
R. L. Slayton, E. A. Palmer, *Traumatic Dental Injuries in Children*,
https://doi.org/10.1007/978-3-030-25793-4_9

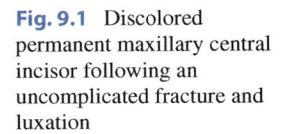

Fig. 9.1 Discolored permanent maxillary central incisor following an uncomplicated fracture and luxation

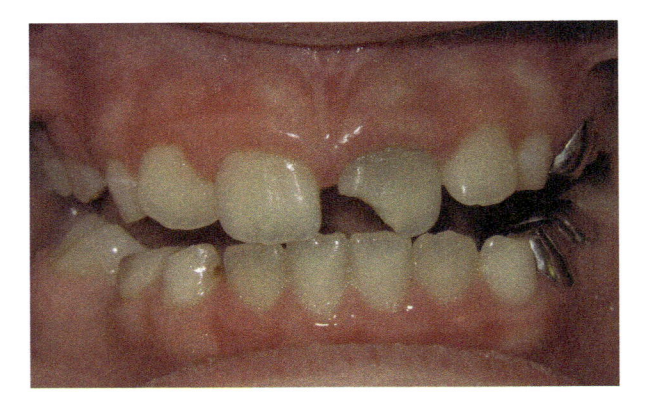

mobility, pain, or inflammatory root resorption before proceeding with endodontic treatment on a traumatized primary tooth. If a primary tooth becomes discolored as a result of an injury, more frequent follow-up evaluations may be indicated due to the increased likelihood of the tooth developing pulpal necrosis.

9.2   Pulpal Necrosis

For a tooth that has developed a reversible pulpitis in response to an injury, it is important to address the cause. Otherwise, the tooth could develop irreversible pulpitis and eventual necrosis. A necrotic pulp is most often due to a complicated crown fracture resulting in an exposed pulp or a luxation injury that interrupts the blood supply and causes pulpal tissue ischemia [2, 7]. Interestingly, while an intrusion injury often causes pulpal necrosis in a permanent tooth, an intruded primary tooth often continues to be vital [8].

A tooth should be monitored closely following an injury because its pulp may not undergo necrosis for several months. A necrotic tooth may not exhibit any clinical or radiographic symptoms other than no response to pulpal vitality testing. However, clinical symptoms of an acute infection could develop, so the tooth should receive appropriate treatment once it is diagnosed with pulpal necrosis.

9.2.1   Treatment of a Nonvital Primary Tooth

The treatment recommended for a primary tooth that has developed pulpal necrosis includes either extraction or pulpectomy followed by restorative therapy. If considering pulpal and restorative treatment, one must first ensure that the tooth has had minimal root resorption and bone loss. Advanced internal or external root resorption and periapical infection that involves the crypt of the succedaneous tooth are contraindications for primary tooth pulpectomy [8]. The dentist should also consider the child's ability to cooperate for treatment in the clinic and if advanced behavior guidance techniques including immobilization, sedation, or general anesthesia would be required. These techniques are discussed in more detail in Chap. 2. A single extraction of a necrotic anterior tooth completed in the dental office may be the treatment of choice for a very young (e.g., 2 years old) child with no other treatment needs. Conversely, an older nervous child (e.g., 5 years old) may be able to sit in the dental chair and cooperate for a longer treatment time so the pulpectomy and restoration may be performed. Or if the child is unable to cooperate for treatment in the clinic, but has extensive needs, he/she may receive comprehensive dental treatment, including the pulpectomy and restoration, under general anesthesia.

9.2.2 Treatment of a Nonvital Immature Permanent Tooth

For a permanent tooth with a necrotic pulp, the treatment options are based on the maturity of the tooth. An immature necrotic tooth with incomplete root formation and an open apex presents a treatment challenge. As a nonvital immature tooth is prone to root resorption, treatment of the root canal should proceed as soon as possible. However, with the thin dentinal wall and wide-open apex, it is difficult to deliver gutta-percha condensed in the area. Apexification therapy has historically been the treatment of choice in this instance in order to use a medicament (often calcium hydroxide) to induce the formation of a hard tissue barrier at the apex [9]. One of the challenges with apexification is that it is a multiple step process, and the patient must return for multiple visits over a 3- to 21-month time span in order to monitor the tooth for apical closure [10]. Additionally, there is opportunity for the canal to become reinfected due to leakage around the temporary coronal filling and thereby compromising the apexification process.

The apical barrier technique was developed as an alternative to apexification because it allows for the comprehensive root canal therapy to be performed in a shorter time duration. In the apical barrier technique, the canals are disinfected with irrigants and instrumentation. Mineral trioxide aggregate (MTA) is then placed in the apical one-third of the canal. The canal is filled and a permanent restoration is placed. The goal of the MTA apical plug is not only to create an apical barrier with which to condense root filling against, but to also induce root end closure at the apex. One challenge with this process is that the roots still remain thin and fragile with a higher risk of fracture and tooth loss [11].

Regenerative endodontics is a paradigm shift in the treatment of nonvital immature teeth that allows for continued root maturation and apical closure [12–14]. Regenerative endodontics procedures remove damaged and diseased tissue and replace them with viable, immunocompetent tissue inside the root canal which can restore the biological structure and functions of the dental pulp. Thus root length and thickness should increase thereby minimizing fragility [11]. The process of regenerative endodontics includes two steps. First, the root canal system is disinfected with minimal or no instrumentation, irrigation with sodium hypochlorite and EDTA, and may include the application of an intracanal medicament such as calcium hydroxide or an antibiotic paste. Second, at a subsequent appointment, an instrument is used at the apical tissue to induce bleeding into the canal and create a blood clot. The blood clot is capped with MTA or biodentine, and the tooth is restored. The majority of providers complete these steps in two visits; however, there are cases reported demonstrating single visit success [15, 16]. The outcome measures for regenerative endodontics are similar to that of other treatment techniques and include absence of signs and symptoms of inflammation and radiographic evidence of resolution of periapical lesions. Additionally, a tooth that is treated with regenerative endodontics should also demonstrate increased root length and canal wall thickness as well as a positive response to pulpal sensibility testing. Two recent systematic reviews demonstrated 91% success rates with regenerative endodontics procedures with 80% success in increased root development and 76% success in apical closure [17, 18].

9.2.3 Treatment of a Nonvital Mature Permanent Tooth

A nonvital permanent tooth with complete root development and apical closure would traditionally undergo conventional endodontic therapy. However, there are reports in the literature of the successful performance of regenerative endodontics treatment of mature permanent teeth [19, 20]. While the data is minimal given the limited studies currently available, the potential to be able to regenerate the pulpal tissue of both mature and immature permanent teeth would be a significant shift in endodontic treatment approaches.

9.3 Pulp Canal Obliteration

Pulp canal obliteration (PCO) is the process of excessive and rapid dentin apposition due to pulpal healing in response to a traumatic dental injury (TDI) [21]. PCO is most often associated with teeth with open apices that experience extrusion or lateral luxation injuries [22–26]. For a tooth undergoing PCO, the coronal pulp chamber and canal space will decrease in size until it may radiographically appear not to exist (Fig. 9.2); however, the obliteration is not complete. There is an extremely narrow root canal containing pulpal tissue. Not surprisingly, clinical reports have demonstrated a reduction in response to thermal and electrical pulp testing as the PCO becomes more pronounced [27]. With the excessive deposition of dentin, a tooth that has gone through PCO may appear a yellowish or grayish opaque color (Fig. 9.3).

The process of PCO does not seem to alter a primary tooth's ability to go through normal root resorption and exfoliation. For permanent teeth, 1–27.5% develop apical periodontitis and pulpal necrosis as a late complication following PCO [22, 27]. The diagnosis of pulpal necrosis must be based on periapical changes noted on the radiographic images instead of sensibility testing and discoloration [22, 27]. Because the frequency of pulpal necrosis in traumatized permanent teeth with PCO is low, prophylactic endodontic therapy of a tooth with PCO is not indicated. Instead, regular, long-term clinical and radiographic follow-up should be implemented [21].

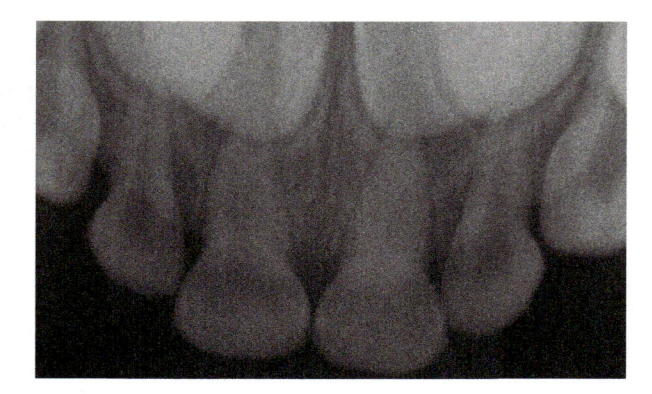

Fig. 9.2 Pulp canal obliteration (PCO) evident in an occlusal radiograph of a primary left maxillary central incisor. There are no signs of pulp necrosis but regular clinical and radiographic evaluation is recommended. (Courtesy of Dr. Travis Nelson)

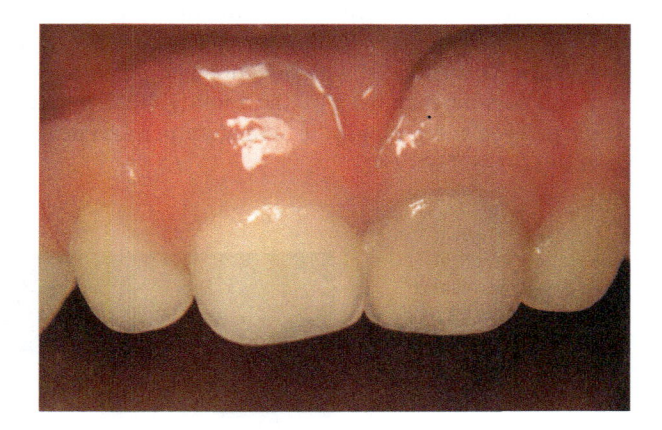

Fig. 9.3 Discolored primary left maxillary incisor due to pulp canal obliteration (PCO). There are no clinical or radiographic signs of pulp necrosis. (Courtesy of Dr. Travis Nelson)

9.4 Inflammatory Resorption

Traumatic injuries (such as lateral luxation, intrusion, and avulsion) to the dentition that damage the PDL and cause neurovascular disruption are most often associated with the development of inflammatory resorption. Inflammatory resorption is a phenomenon in which odontoclasts cause a significant amount of damage to the cementum, dentin, and/or bone. It can present as either internal or external resorption of the root, with external resorption being more frequent [28, 29].

9.4.1 Internal Inflammatory Resorption

Internal inflammatory resorption is a relatively rare response to trauma. Transiently, it may involve only the loss of the odontoblast layer and the predentin within an area of the canal surface and is considered self-limiting. However, if the pulp tissue is contaminated by bacteria, then the odontoclasts' resorption process progresses and affects the internal dentin surface of the tooth. Internal inflammatory resorption requires vital tissue at the site of the resorptive defect, the section of the pulp coronal to the defect may be necrotic. Internal inflammatory resorption continues until the pulp tissue is necrotic. Unfortunately, at that point, severe damage may have already ensued thereby compromising the tooth [29–31].

9.4.2 External Inflammatory Resorption

External inflammatory resorption is characterized by bowl-shaped areas of resorption that begin in the periodontium and involve the cementum and dentin of the tooth. While transient external inflammatory resorption may be self-limited to the cementoblasts and cementum of the tooth, progressive external inflammatory resorption involving the dentin may advance quickly. This type of resorption is almost always associated with infection and pulp necrosis and should be managed with endodontic treatment of the tooth [30]. External inflammatory resorption develops even more rapidly in immature permanent teeth than those with closed apices [32–34] (Fig. 9.4).

Fig. 9.4 External resorption of permanent mandibular incisors following replantation and delayed root canal treatment

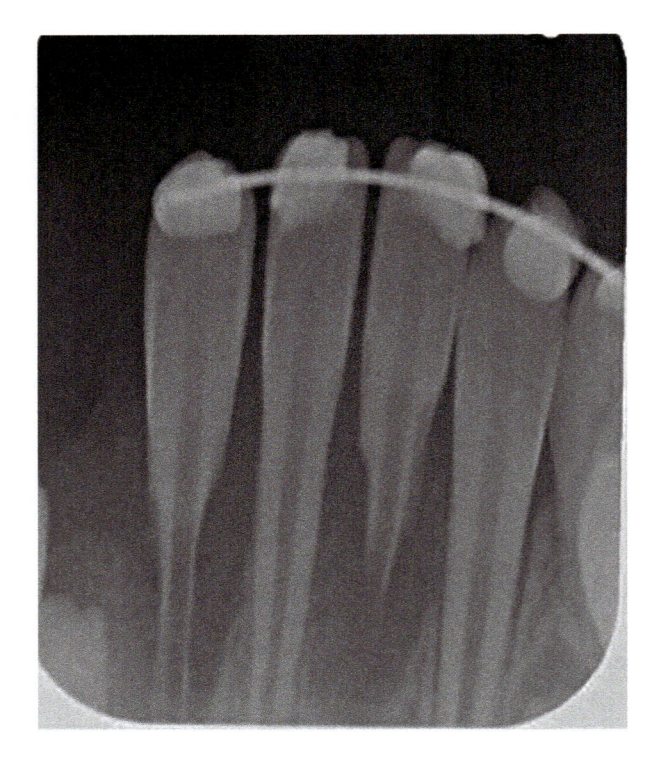

9.4.3   Treatment Recommendations

Both internal and external inflammatory resorption are most often diagnosed within the first 2–3 years after an injury has occurred, but in some instances, root resorption can be visualized at 21 days following the trauma [34, 35]. Teeth undergoing inflammatory resorption are usually asymptomatic. Thus, it is important to closely monitor patients that have suffered from dental trauma for the development of inflammatory resorption. As soon as the inflammatory resorption process in a permanent tooth is visualized radiographically, endodontic root canal therapy must occur as soon as possible [35, 36]. After removal of the pulpal tissue and irrigation of the canals, calcium hydroxide is then often placed in order to create an environment that is antibacterial [35, 37]. The calcium hydroxide may be replaced if the resorptive process continues. Once radiographic confirmation of the cessation of the process is obtained, then the canal(s) is filled with gutta-percha and the tooth is restored. In cases of extreme inflammatory resorption, extraction may be the only option.

9.5   Ankylosis/Replacement Resorption

Replacement resorption (ankylosis) is most commonly observed after trauma to the anterior primary or permanent teeth in response to severe luxation injuries like avulsions or intrusions in which the PDL cells are damaged and thus induces an inflammatory process. The cementum comes in direct contact with the bone. The osteoclastic cells from the remodeling bone resorb areas of the contacting cementum, the root surface tissue is progressively replaced with bone, and the tissues become fused. Replacement resorption typically proceeds more quickly in a child or adolescent because of the increased rate of physiologic bone remodeling in comparison to an adult [38].

An ankylosed tooth is unable to respond to the continual eruptive process as the other teeth do, and thus will be in infraocclusion (Fig. 9.5). The degree by which the infraocclusion presents can vary from a mild infraocclusion limited to the ankylosed tooth and adjacent bone to a severe presentation in which the alveolar ridge has an unaesthetic deficiency and the adjacent teeth may tip into the ankylosed tooth. The severity of infraocclusion is more pronounced when the replacement resorption process is initiated in children and adolescents who are still growing. Replacement resorption can also be diagnosed clinically because the ankylosed tooth lacks normal physiologic mobility. Additionally, an ankylosed tooth will have a metallic percussion sound [39]. Radiographically, the resorbed areas of root have been replaced with bone, and the PDL space is not visible; however, ankylotic areas of a root surface will only be visible radiographically if at least 20% of the root surface is affected [40].

Fig. 9.5 Ankylosis of permanent right maxillary central incisor demonstrated by infraposition relative to the contralateral incisor. Treatment options include decoronation and extraction

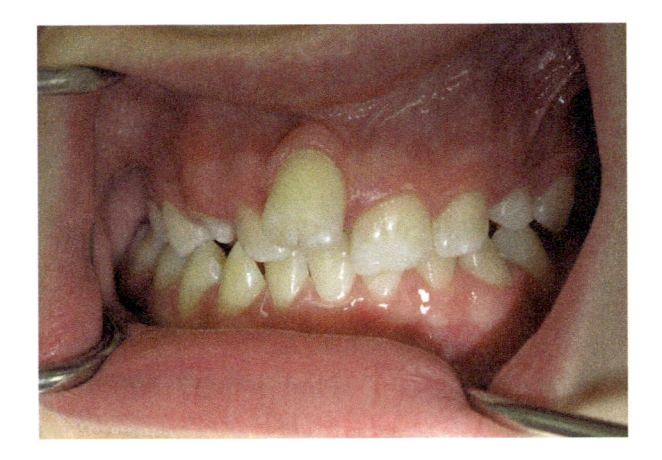

9.5.1 Treatment of Ankylosed Primary Teeth

The development of replacement resorption in a primary tooth as a sequelae of previous trauma, is very rare [41, 42]. A recent retrospective study reported that it occurs in 3.6% of previously intruded primary teeth and 1.4% of previously laterally luxated primary teeth [41, 43]. In all of these cases, the ankylosed tooth had been treated by extraction. However, there is very little research about how an ankylosed primary tooth following trauma should optimally be treated. The relationship between the ankylosed tooth and the successor permanent tooth's bud should be evaluated on a case-by-case basis, and the ankylosed primary incisor should be extracted if it appears to be inhibiting permanent tooth development and/or eruption [41].

9.5.2 Treatment of Ankylosed Permanent Teeth

Ankylosis of a permanent tooth may pose several treatment challenges to a dental provider. This is especially true in a growing child or adolescent in whom the replacement root resorption rate is rapid as is the child's growth and development. In this instance, the degree of infraocclusion may be more severe. As the process of replacement resorption is progressive and there are not currently any treatment modalities by which to stop or reverse it, if no treatment is employed, the entire root will be replaced by bone and the crown will fall off or be removed [44]. Thus, several treatment modalities have historically been employed in order to address an ankylosed tooth including surgical luxation, orthodontic distraction, autotransplantation, composite build-ups, or extraction followed by implant placement [38, 45, 46]. Most recently, decoronation and replacement root resorption has become an alternative treatment of choice for an ankylosed permanent tooth [47].

Fig. 9.6 Ankylosis of both permanent maxillary central incisors (**a**) resulting from avulsion and replantation. Decoronation was initiated (**b**). (Courtesy of the University of Iowa Department of Pediatric Dentistry)

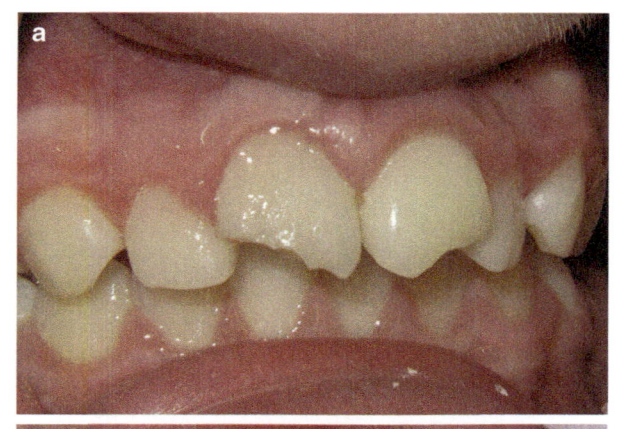
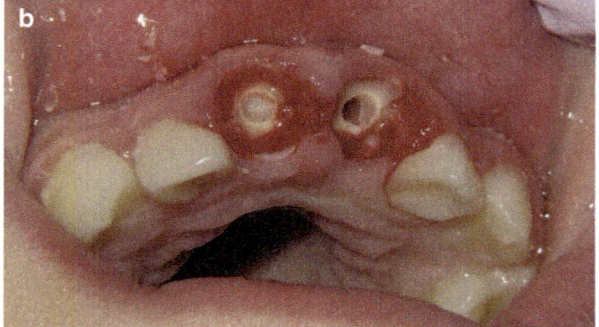

Decoronation is the process in which an ankylosed tooth crown is removed while the resorbing root becomes a scaffold for new alveolar bone deposition. An ankylosed tooth first undergoes a coronectomy below the level of the cementoenamel junction (CEJ) (Fig. 9.6a, b). Second, any root filling material is removed, and then the periapical area of the pulp is instrumented in order to stimulate bleeding (Fig. 9.7a). The coronal surface of the root is then covered with a mucoperiosteal flap [38, 47] (Fig. 9.7b). Depending on the age and developmental stage of the patient, a fixed or removable appliance may be employed as a temporary restoration following a decoronation procedure. The patient may then have an implant placed upon completion of their growth.

Decoronation has been demonstrated to maintain, and even enhance, the height and width of the alveolar ridge so that an implant may be placed in the future with a better esthetic outcome [48–51]. However, the alveolar bone has been demonstrated to increase, most significantly in patients that are treated prior to their pubertal growth [38, 44]. Malmgren and colleagues followed patients that had undergone decoronation procedures as adolescents. They found that males at a mean age of 14.6 years and females at a mean age of 13 years at the time of the decoronation procedure experienced the most favorable increase in bone levels. Conversely,

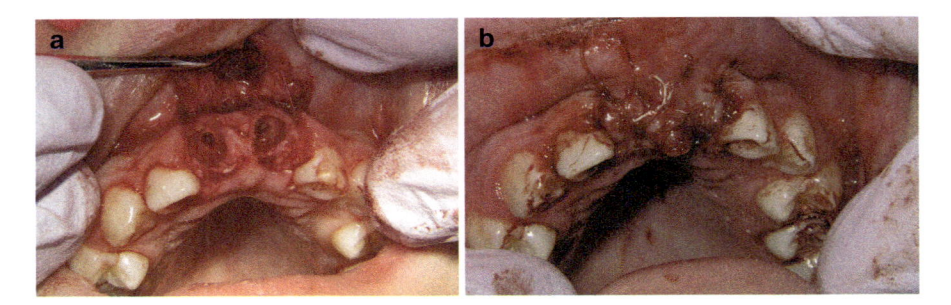

Fig. 9.7 As part of the decoronation procedure, a flap was laid and tooth structure was removed below the alveolar ridge (**a**). An endodontic file is used to bring blood and cells from the apex of the tooth into the root canal. The final step of decoronation involves suturing the flap over the roots to create a seal (**b**)

decoronation procedures carried out in individuals after the age of 16 years resulted in either an unchanged or reduced alveolar bone level [44].

In order to minimize unaesthetic outcomes, a tooth that has undergone an avulsion, lateral luxation, or intrusion injury should be monitored closely long-term. Thus, a tooth undergoing replacement resorption (ankylosis) will be identified and addressed as soon as possible. This will allow for a minimal discrepancy in infraocclusion as well as will allow for the decoronated tooth to resorb and serve as a matrix for maximal alveolar bone growth.

9.6 Premature Loss of Primary Tooth

A primary tooth that has experienced a traumatic dental injury may be prematurely lost as a result of avulsion, extraction due to the poor prognosis as a result of the injury, late complications following the injury, or premature exfoliation due to accelerated root resorption [52]. The premature loss of a primary incisor can affect esthetics, eating, speech development, oral habit development, arch integrity, and quality of life [52]. Additionally, because the child may have limited ability to cooperate for in office treatment, the fabrication of a temporary appliance in order to replace the missing tooth may not be practical. Given that the loss of a primary tooth is expected at some point, its premature loss may not be recognized by a dental provider as being as negative of an outcome as if it had been a permanent tooth. However, to the family, the sudden change in the child's smile may be very dramatic. It is very important to thoroughly communicate with the family and to assuage their concerns. Stressing the transient nature and the inevitability of missing teeth during childhood may help the family to adjust to the change. It is also important to make families aware that the premature loss of a primary incisor frequently results in delayed eruption of the permanent successor. They should not be alarmed if the contralateral tooth erupts earlier than the tooth whose predecessor was lost prematurely.

9.7 Damage to the Succedaneous Tooth by the Injured Primary Tooth

One potentially severe sequela of a traumatic injury to a primary tooth is a developmental disturbance in the succedaneous tooth. Anatomically, the permanent successor tooth develops in close proximity to the apex of the primary tooth [1, 53]. Thus, a primary tooth that undergoes a traumatic injury or the development of a periapical lesion associated with pulpal necrosis could lead to damage of the adjacent developing succedaneous tooth.

The severity of the injury and the age of the child both play a role in whether or not a developmental disturbance and thus damage occurs to the succedaneous tooth.

With an increase in the severity of the primary tooth injury, the probability for the development of a disturbance increases. While subluxation injuries in primary teeth have been reported to cause damage to the permanent successor in 10–34% of cases, intrusion and avulsion injuries have been reported to cause damage in 40–70% and 30–50% of the cases, respectively [53–59]. The age of the patient at the time of the injury is also associated with the presence and severity of the damage. Developmental disturbances were identified in 94.5% of permanent successor teeth when avulsion of their primary predecessors occurred in children up to age 2 years, 80% of succedaneous teeth in children aged 2–4 years, and 18.2% after 5 years old [60]. Thus, it is important to consider the potential damage to the permanent tooth when addressing a primary tooth injury, and treatment decisions should be focused on minimizing the potential negative sequelae.

Types of developmental disturbances observed as sequelae in permanent successors include enamel defects, crown and root dilacerations, and altered eruption timing or direction.

9.7.1 Enamel Defects

If the primary tooth injury occurs during the permanent crown formation, a developmental disturbance of the enamel may occur. The different types of observed enamel defects as a result of trauma include enamel discoloration (Fig. 9.8a), opacity (Fig. 9.8b), hypoplasia and hypomineralization. Enamel discoloration and/or hypoplasia are the most common of all of the developmental disturbances due to primary tooth dental trauma [53, 55–57, 60–62]. This is thought to be because the maturation of mineralized enamel continues until the tooth erupts even though the crown formation of a permanent incisor is complete when a child is 3 years old [53, 62]. Additionally, the predominance of enamel defects as opposed to other disturbances is thought to be because they can result from less severe trauma to primary incisors [63].

Enamel defects can cause compromised esthetics, tooth sensitivity, increased risk for caries, and tooth wear. Depending on the severity and type of the enamel defect, varying treatment will be indicated. Enamel defects should be documented and photographed to aid in accurate diagnosis, treatment planning, and follow-up.

Fig. 9.8 Traumatic injuries to primary teeth may result in enamel defects in the permanent successors including yellow (**a**) or white (**b**) opacities. These defects may put the tooth at increased risk for caries and are an esthetic concern as well

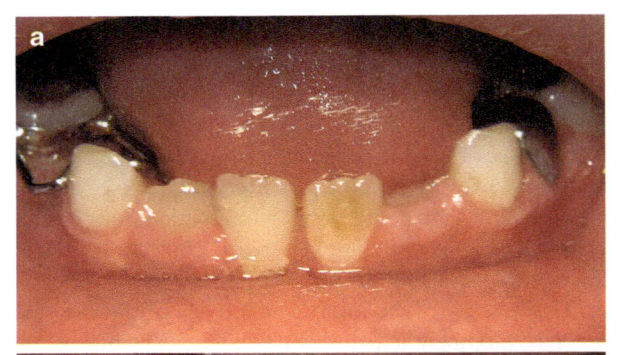

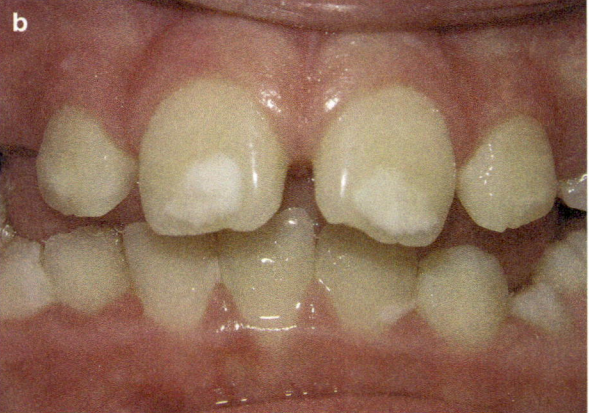

To reduce the caries risk, professional fluoride applications every 3–6 months should be encouraged and the importance of excellent oral hygiene at home should be stressed. Mild discoloration, hypoplasia, and/or opacities may be initially approached conservatively. Enamel microabrasion with or without at home bleaching has also been demonstrated to successfully treat enamel discoloration, hypoplasia, and opacities [64–68]. Resin infiltration is a minimally invasive technique that has also shown success in the treatment of enamel defects [69–71] (Fig. 9.9a, b). If the conservative treatment options are not successful, or in the cases of severe enamel defects, direct composite resin restorations, composite resin or porcelain veneers, or full coverage crowns may be indicated.

9.7.2   Crown and Root Dilaceration

A dilacerated crown or root has an abnormal angulation or curvature in respect to the rest of the tooth. A dilaceration may occur during a traumatic injury if the primary tooth displaces the already calcified portion of the developing succedaneous tooth while the remainder of the tooth continues to form with an abnormal

Fig. 9.9 Enamel defects on the facial of both permanent maxillary central incisors (**a**). Appearance of incisors after resin infiltration (Icon®—DMG America) (**b**). (Courtesy of Dr. Richard Chaet)

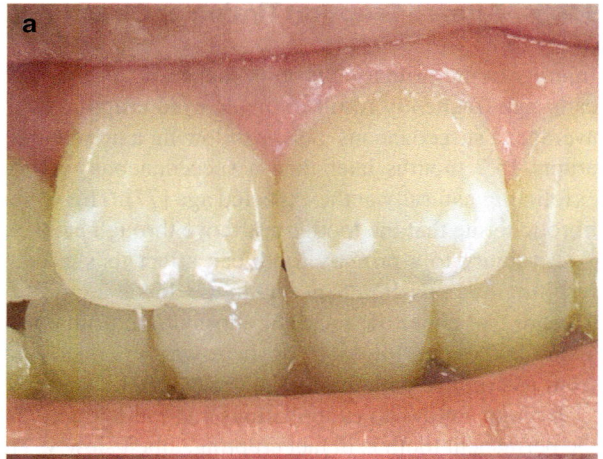

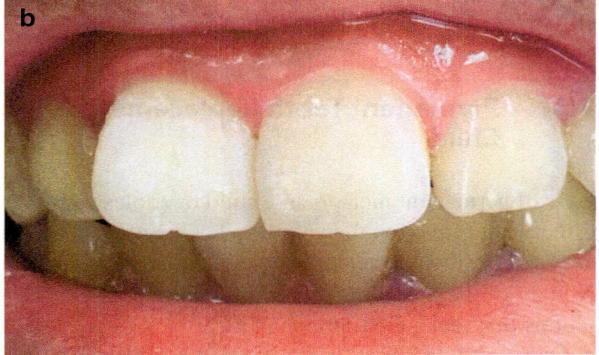

angle [72]. Dilacerations are most often associated with intrusions and avulsions of primary teeth and most often affect the mandibular and maxillary central incisors. About half of these teeth are impacted and can cause midline deviations and mesial angulation of adjacent teeth. Crown and root dilacerations have been reported to result in 10–13% and 1–17%, respectively, cases of trauma to primary teeth [1, 54, 72–75]. Whether the crown or the root becomes dilacerated is associated with the age of the child at the time of the injury. A dilacerated crown is more often the sequelae in a child injured at age 4 years or younger, while a root dilaceration is more often the result in a child over the age of 4 years [1, 73, 76].

Treatment of a tooth with a dilaceration can be complex. An impacted tooth with a dilacerated crown or root may be either extracted or surgically exposed and orthodontically extruded. If the tooth has erupted or has been orthodontically extruded, the crown may be resected, a root canal performed, and a restoration placed.

9.7.3   Altered Eruption Timing or Direction

Injuries to the primary dentition that result in the loss of the primary tooth at an early age frequently result in the delayed eruption of the permanent successor. On average, a succedaneous incisor following a prematurely exfoliated primary incisor erupts 15.7 months later than a succedaneous tooth replacing a primary incisor exfoliating naturally at the expected age [77]. This is thought to be due to additional fibrotic tissue that the tooth must move through at an extraction or avulsion site.

An injury to a primary tooth can affect its succedaneous tooth's eruption path resulting in a misalignment within the dental arch. Possible reasons for this alteration are that either the premature loss of the primary tooth leads to a lack of guidance for the erupting tooth or there was a deflection of the developing tooth bud from its eruptive path during the trauma [62].

Regular follow-up examinations and radiographs should be taken to ensure that the permanent tooth is in fact erupting, albeit slowly. The malalignment can then be corrected orthodontically.

9.8   Permanent Tooth Replacement Options in the Growing Child

Loss of permanent incisors in a child or adolescent who is still growing, presents an esthetic and functional challenge. There are a number of ways to replace teeth that are esthetically acceptable, including temporary fixed or removable partial dentures. Neither of these options preserve alveolar bone height or width and both have limitations that make them less than ideal.

9.8.1   Temporary Partial Dentures

A removable partial denture, sometimes referred to as a "flipper" is similar to an orthodontic retainer with acrylic on the palate, clasps on molars for retention and one or more acrylic teeth designed to match the shade and shape of the natural teeth as closely as possible. These appliances have the disadvantage of being easily lost or broken, relatively expensive, and not always covered by insurance. Children with developmental disorders or sensory issues may find this appliance very difficult to tolerate.

A temporary fixed partial denture is fabricated by fitting orthodontic bands on the permanent first molars, making an impression and sending the impression or stone model to the laboratory. The partial is designed with an archwire along the palatal surfaces of the maxillary teeth with an acrylic button in the anterior region and an acrylic tooth attached to the acrylic button. This appliance can provide improved esthetics, is often less expensive than a removable partial denture, and does not have the risk of being lost since it is cemented onto the molars. One disadvantage is that is at risk for breaking, especially if the child has a traumatic injury or bites into hard or chewy food. For this type of appliance, it is also necessary for the child to be able to cooperate for band fitting, impressions, and cementation of the appliance.

9.8.2 Autotransplantation

A third option for replacement of missing incisors is autotransplantation. This is a well-documented procedure that involves extracting a donor tooth (often a premolar) and transplanting it into the site of the missing permanent incisor. This method and details of the indications for its use are described in detail by Andreasen et al. [78] and will be briefly discussed here.

Advantages of autotransplantation are that it can be performed in a growing child. Unlike the temporary partial dentures described above, autotransplantation preserves alveolar bone and helps create new alveolar bone [78]. The long-term prognosis and esthetics are similar to that of implants, but implants aren't indicated for adolescents who are still growing. Donor teeth (also referred to as grafts) should be considered based on their crown and root anatomy. For maxillary central incisors, the most suitable donor teeth are second mandibular premolars, canines, first mandibular premolars, and second maxillary premolars [78]. In some cases, very small third molars may be used.

Success of an autotransplantation procedure is more likely when the donor tooth has three-fourths to full root development with an open apex, the surgical extraction is done non-traumatically and there is adequate bone support for the donor tooth [78, 79]. Mature teeth can also be successfully transplanted but generally require root canal treatment, as pulp regeneration is unlikely in these teeth.

In a study of autotransplantation in children and adolescents, Kafourou et al. demonstrated that pulp and PDL healing occurred in all immature donor teeth. In mature teeth, 77% had favorable PDL healing and 22% had favorable pulp healing [79]. In this sample, overall success of transplantation was 87.6%.

The success of this procedure also depends on multiple experienced specialists working together. In most cases, the team consists of an oral surgeon, prosthodontist, endodontist, orthodontist, pediatric dentist, and/or general dentist. Depending on the age and ability of the child to tolerate the procedure, general anesthesia may be necessary.

References

1. Andreasen JO, Andreasen FM, Andersson L. Textbook and color atlas of traumatic injuries to the teeth. 5th ed. Hoboken: Wiley-Blackwell; 2019. p. 377–412.
2. Andreasen FM, Pedersen BV. Prognosis of luxated permanent teeth – the development of pulp necrosis. Endod Dent Traumatol. 1985;1:207–20.
3. Andreasen FM, Yu Z, Thomsen BL. Relationship between pulp dimensions and development of pulp necrosis after luxation injuries in the permanent dentition. Endod Dent Traumatol. 1986;2:90–8.

4. Croll TP, Pascon EA, Langeland K. Traumatically injured primary incisors; a clinical and histological study. ASDC J Dent Child. 1987;54:401–22.
5. Holan G, Fuks AB. The diagnostic value of coronal dark-gray discoloration in primary teeth following traumatic injuries. Pediatr Dent. 1996;18:224–7.
6. Cardoso M, Rocha MJ. Association of crown discoloration and pulp status in traumatized primary teeth. Dent Traumatol. 2010;26:413–6.
7. Robertson A, Andreasen FM, Andreasen JO, Norén JG. Long-term prognosis of crown-fractured permanent incisors: the effect of stage of root development and associated luxation injury. Int J Paediatr Dent. 2000;10:191–9.
8. Holan G, McTigue DJ. Introduction to dental trauma: Managing traumatic injuries in the primary dentition. In: Nowak AJ, Christensen JR, Mabry TR, Townsend JA, Wells MH, editors. Pediatric dentistry infancy through adolescence. Philadelphia: Elsevier; 2019. p. 227–43.
9. Simon S, Rilliard F, Berdal A, Machtou P. The use of mineral trioxide aggregate in one visit apexification treatment: A prospective study. Int Endod J. 2007;40:186–97.
10. Giuliani V, Baccetti T, Pace R, Pagavino G. The use of MTA in teeth with necrotic pulps and open apices. Dent Traumatol. 2002;18:217–21.
11. Galler KM. Clinical procedures for revitalization: current knowledge and considerations. Int Endod J. 2016;49:926–36.
12. Chueh LH, Huang GT. Immature teeth with periradicular periodontitis or abscess undergoing apexogenesis: a paradigm shift. J Endod. 2006;32:1205–13.
13. Huang GT. A paradigm shift in endodontic management of immature teeth: conservation of stem cells for regeneration. J Dent. 2008;36:379–86.
14. Huang GT, Sonoyama W, Liu Y, Liu H, Wang S, Shi S. The hidden treasure in apical papilla: the potential role in pulp/dentin regeneration and bioroot engineering. J Endod. 2008;34:645–51.
15. Shin SY, Albert JS, Mortman RE. One step pulp revascularization treatment of an immature permanent tooth with chronic apical abscess: a case report. Int Endod J. 2009;42:1118–26.
16. McCabe P. Revascularization of an immature tooth with apical periodontitis using a single visit protocol: a case report. Int Endod J. 2015;48:484–97.
17. Tong HJ, Rajan S, Bhujel N, Kang J, Duggal M, Nazzal H. Regenerative endodontic therapy in the management of nonvital immature permanent teeth: a systematic review-outcome evaluation and meta-analysis. J Endod. 2017;43:1453–64.
18. Torabinejad M, Nosrat A, Verma P, Udochukwu O. Regenerative endodontic treatment or mineral trioxide aggregate apical plug in teeth with necrotic pulps and open apices: a systematic review and meta-analysis. J Endod. 2017;43:1806–20.
19. Paryani K, Kim SG. Regenerative endodontic treatment of permanent teeth after completion of root development: a report of 2 cases. J Endod. 2013;39:929–34.
20. Saoud TM, Martin G, Chen YH, Chen KL, Chen CA, Songtrakul K. Treatment of mature permanent teeth with necrotic pulps and apical periodontitis using regenerative endodontic procedures: a case series. J Endod. 2016;42:57–65.
21. Bastos JV, Côrtes MI. Pulp canal obliteration after traumatic injuries in permanent teeth – scientific fact or fiction? Braz Oral Res. 2018;32:e75. https://doi.org/10.1590/1807-3107bor-2018.vol32.0075.
22. Andreasen FM, Zhijie Y, Thomsen BL, Andersen PK. Occurrence of pulp canal obliteration after luxation injuries in the permanent dentition. Endod Dent Traumatol. 1987;3:103–15.
23. Oikarinen K, Gundlach KK, Pfeifer G. Late complications of luxation injuries to teeth. Endod Dent Traumatol. 1987;3:296–303.
24. Lee R, Barrett EJ, Kenny DJ. Clinical outcomes for permanent incisor luxations in a pediatric population. II. Extrusions. Dent Traumatol. 2003;1:274–9.
25. Nikoui M, Kenny DJ, Barrett EJ. Clinical outcomes for permanent incisor luxations in a pediatric population. III. Lateral luxations. Dent Traumatol. 2003;19:280–5.
26. Hecova J, Tzigkounakis V, Merglova V, Netolicky J. A retrospective study of 889 injured permanent teeth. Dent Traumatol. 2010;26:466–75.
27. Oginni AO, Adekoya-Sofowora CA, Kolawole KA. Evaluation of radiographs, clinical signs and symptoms associated with pulp canal obliteration: an aid to treatment decision. Dent Traumatol. 2009;25:620–5.

28. Tronstad L. Root resorption: etiology, terminology and clinical manifestations. Endod Dent Traumatol. 1988;4:241–52.
29. Patel S, Ricucci D, Durak C, Tay F. Internal root resorption: a review. J Endod. 2010;36:1107–21.
30. Wedenberg C, Lindskop S. Experimental internal resorption in monkey teeth. Endod Dent Traumatol. 1985;1:221–7.
31. Wedenberg C, Lindskog S. Evidence for a resorption inhibitor in dentine. Eur J Oral Sci. 1987;95:205–11.
32. Soares AJ, Gomes BPFA, Zaia AA, Ferraz CCR, Souza-Filho FJ. Relationship between clinical-radiographic evaluation and outcome of teeth replantation. Dent Traumatol. 2008;24:183–8.
33. Kinirons MJ, Gregg TA, Welbury RR, Cole BOI. Variations in the presenting and treatment features in reimplanted permanent incisors in children and their effect on the prevalence of root resorption. Br Dent J. 2000;189:263–6.
34. Soares AJ, Souza GA, Pereira AC, Vargas-Neto J, Zaia AA, Silva EJNL. Frequency of root resorption following trauma to permanent teeth. J Oral Sci. 2015;57:73–8.
35. Andreasen JO, Borum MK, Jacobsen HL, Andreasen FM. Replantation of 400 avulsed permanent incisors. 4. Factors related to periodontal ligament healing. Endod Dent Traumatol. 1995;11:76–89.
36. Souza BDM, Dutra KL, Kuntze MM, Bortoluzzi EA, Flores-Mir C, Reyes-Carmona J, Felippe WT, Porporatti AL, De Luca Canto G. Incidence of root resorption after the replantation of avulsed teeth: a meta-analysis. J Endod. 2018;44:1216–27.
37. Sjögren U, Figdor D, Spångberg L, Sundqvist G. The antimicrobial effect of calcium hydroxide as a short-term intracanal dressing. Int Endod J. 1991;24:119–25.
38. Mohadeb JVN, Somar M, He H. Effectiveness of decoronation technique in the treatment of ankyloses: a systematic review. Dent Traumatol. 2016;32:255–63.
39. Fuss Z, Tsesis I, Lin S. Root resorption – diagnosis, classification and treatment choices based on stimulation factors. Dent Traumatol. 2003;19:175–82.
40. Andersson L, Blomlöf L, Lindskog S, Feiglin B, Hammarström L. Tooth ankyloses. Clinical, radiographic and histological assessment. Int J Oral Surg. 1984;13:423–31.
41. Lauridsen E, Blanche P, Yousaf N, Andreasen JO. The risk of healing complications in primary teeth with intrusive luxation-a retrospective cohort study. Dent Traumatol. 2017;33:329–36.
42. Borym MK, Andreasen JO. Sequelae of trauma to primary maxillary incisors. I. Complications in the primary dentition. Endod Dent Traumatol. 1998;14:31–44.
43. Lauridsen E, Blanche P, Yousaf N, Andreasen JO. The risk of healing complications in primary teeth with extrusive or lateral luxation-a retrospective cohort study. Dent Traumatol. 2017;33:307–16.
44. Malmgren B, Tsilingaridis G, Malmgren O. Long-term follow up of 103 ankylosed permanent incisors surgically treated with decoronation – a retrospective cohort study. Dent Traumatol. 2015;31:184–9.
45. Andersson L, Malmgren B. The problem of dentoalveolar ankyloses and subsequent replacement resorption in the growing patient. Aust Endod J. 1999;25:57–61.
46. Stanford N. Treatment of ankylosed permanent teeth. Evid Based Dent. 2010;11:44.
47. Malmgren B, Cvek M, Lundberg M, Frykholm A. Surgical treatment of ankylosed and infrapositioned reimplanted incisors in adolescents. Scand J Dent Res. 1984;92:391–9.
48. Lin S, Schwarz-Arad D, Ashkenazi M. Alveolar bone width preservation after decoronation of ankylosed anterior incisors. J Endod. 2013;39:1542–4.
49. Sapir S, Kalter A, Sapir MR. Decoronation of an ankylosed permanent incisor: alveolar ridge preservation and rehabilitation by an implant supported porcelain crown. Dent Traumatol. 2009;25:346–9.
50. Cohenca N, Stabholz A. Decoronation – a conservative method to treat ankylosed teeth for preservation of alveolar ridge prior to permanent prosthetic reconstruction: literature review and case presentation. Dent Traumatol. 2007;23:87–94.
51. Malmgren B, Malmgren O, Andreasen JO. Alveolar bone development after decoronation of ankylosed teeth. Endod Topics. 2006;14:35–40.
52. Holan G, Needleman HL. Premature loss of primary anterior teeth due to trauma – potential short- and long-term sequelae. Dent Traumatol. 2014;30:100–6.

53. von Arx T. Developmental disturbances of permanent teeth following trauma to the primary dentition. Aust Dent J. 1993;38:1–10.
54. Andreasen JO, Ravn JJ. The effect of traumatic injuries to primary teeth on their permanent successors. II. A clinical and radiographic follow-up study of 213 teeth. Scand J Dent Res. 1971;79:284–94.
55. Sennhenn-Kirchner S, Jacobs HG. Traumatic injuries to the primary dentition and effects on the permanent successors – a clinical follow-up study. Dent Traumatol. 2006;22:237–41.
56. Assunção LRS, Ferelle A, Iwakura ML, Cunha RF. Effects on permanent teeth after luxation injuries to the primary predecessors: a study in children assisted at the emergency service. Dent Traumatol. 2009;25:165–70.
57. Christophersen P, Freund M, Harild L. Avulsion of primary teeth and sequelae on the permanent successors. Dent Traumatol. 2005;21:320–3.
58. Altun C, Cehreli ZC, Güven G, Acikel C. Traumatic intrusion of primary teeth and its effects on the permanent successors: a clinical follow-up study. Oral Surg Oral Med Oral Pathol Oral Radiol Endod. 2009;107:493–8.
59. Skaare AB, Aas ALM, Wang NJ. Enamel defects in permanent incisors after trauma to primary predecessors: inter-observer agreement based on photographs. Dent Traumatol. 2013;29:79–83.
60. Ravn JJ. Developmental disturbances in permanent teeth after exarticulation of their primary predecessors. Scand J Dent Res. 1975;83:131–4.
61. Carvalho V, Jacomo DR, Campos V. Frequency of intrusion in deciduous teeth and its effects. Dent Traumatol. 2010;26:304–7.
62. Ben-Bassat Y, Brin I, Fuks A, Zilberman Y. Effects of trauma to the primary incisors on permanent successors in different developmental stages. Pediatr Dent. 1985;7:37–40.
63. Lenzi MM, Alexandria AK, Ferreira DMTP, Maia LC. Does trauma in the primary dentition cause sequelae in permanent successors? A systematic review. Dent Traumatol. 2015;31:79–88.
64. Croll TP, Cavanaugh RR. Enamel color modification by controlled hydrochloric acid-pumice abrasion. II. Further examples. Quintessence Int. 1986;17:157–64.
65. Sundfeld RH, Franco LM, Gonçalves RS, de Alexandre RS, Machado LS, Neto DS. Accomplishing esthetics using enamel microabrasion and bleaching-a case report. Oper Dent. 2014;39:223–7.
66. Sundfeld RH, Sundfeld-Neto D, Machado LS, Franco LM, Fagundes TC, Briso AL. Microabrasion in tooth enamel discoloration defects: three cases with long-term follow-ups. J Appl Oral Sci. 2014;22:347–54.
67. Wray A, Welbury R. UK National Clinical Guidelines in Paediatric Dentistry: treatment of intrinsic discoloration in permanent anterior teeth in children and adolescents. Int J Paediatr Dent. 2001;11:309–15.
68. Croll TP, Helpin ML. Enamel microabrasion: a new approach. J Esthet Dent. 2000;12:64–71.
69. Torres CR, Borges AB. Color masking of developmental enamel defects: a case series. Oper Dent. 2015;40:25–33.
70. Alwafi A. Resin infiltration may be considered as a color-masking treatment option for enamel development defects and white spot lesions. J Evid Based Dent Pract. 2017;17:113–5.
71. Mazur M, Westland S, Guerra F, Corridore D, Vichi M, Maruotti A, Nardi GM, Ottolenghi L. Objective and subjective aesthetic performance of icon® treatment for enamel hypomineralization lesions in young adolescents: a retrospective single center study. J Dent. 2018;68:104–8.
72. de Amorim CS, Americano GCA, Moliterno LFM, de Marsillac MWS, Andrade MRTC, Campos V. Frequency of crown and root dilacerations of permanent incisors after dental trauma to their predecessor teeth. Dent Traumatol. 2018;34:401–5.
73. Zilberman Y, Ben-Bassat Y, Lustmann J, Fuks A, Brin I. Effects of trauma to primary incisors on root development of their permanent successors. Pediatr Dent. 1986;8:289–93.
74. Hamasha AA, Al-Khateeb T, Darwazeh A. Prevalence of dilacerations in Jordanian Adults. Int Endod J. 2002;35:910–2.
75. Bodrumlu E, Gunduz K, Avsever H, Cicek E. A retrospective study of the prevalence and characteristics of root dilacerations in a sample of the Turkish population. Oral Radiol. 2013;29:27–32.

76. Maragakis GM. Crown dilacerations of permanent incisors following trauma to their primary predecessors. J Clin Pediatr Dent. 1995;20:49–52.
77. Korf SR. The eruption of permanent central incisors following premature loss of their antecedents. J Dent Child. 1965;32:39–44.
78. Andreasen JO, Andersson L, Tsukiboshi M, Czochrowska EM. Autotransplantation of teeth to the anterior region. In: Andreasen JO, Andreasen FM, Andersson L, editors. Textbook and color atlas of traumatic injuries to the teeth. 5th ed. Hoboken: Wiley-Blackwell; 2019. p. 853–77.
79. Kafourou V, Tong HJ, Day P, Houghton N, Spencer RJ, Duggal M. Outcomes and prognostic factors that influence the success of tooth autotransplantation in children and adolescents. Dent Traumatol. 2017;33:393–9.

Prevention of Traumatic Dental Injuries   10

It is not possible to eliminate traumatic injuries. As children are learning to walk, participating in sports and actively involved in activities of life, there are always risks of injury. There are many things that can be done to decrease the risk or to minimize the severity of injury. Education about how to decrease risks and manage traumatic injuries and in some cases, regulations to support these activities should be endorsed by all health care providers.

10.1   Child-Proofing Homes

The majority of traumatic dental injuries for young children occur at home. This is primarily due to a fall. As children are learning to walk, they are uncoordinated and can easily trip on uneven surfaces or objects that are left on the floor.

To prevent or minimize injuries to children who are learning to walk, remove items from the floor that a child can trip on and avoid having coffee tables with sharp edges that they can hit their face on. Electric outlets should be covered and electrical cords placed in such a way that children can't easily reach them. Caregivers should be reminded that any electrical cords present a potential danger. With the increased use of phones, notebooks, tablets, and video games, there are more charging cords in most households that may be within reach of a toddler. Dangerous items should be stored out of reach of children. Child gates should be used to keep children from falling down stairs. These are all topics that should be discussed with families during routine dental appointments and are part of a process called anticipatory guidance [1].

R. L. Slayton, E. A. Palmer, *Traumatic Dental Injuries in Children*,
https://doi.org/10.1007/978-3-030-25793-4_10

10.2   Sports: Helmets/Mouthguards

School-aged children are more likely to sustain an injury on the playground or in sporting activities although falls and other injuries at home are still a concern. Many, but not all sports recommend that mouthguards be worn during practice as well as in competition. There is solid evidence to support the effectiveness of mouthguards to prevent or reduce the severity of traumatic dental injuries [2]. There is also evidence that compliance with mouthguard use is not consistent and that a number of sports do not require mouthguards even though it is clear that athletes would benefit from their use. For example, mouthguards are not required in basketball or baseball, yet in one study, there were more dental injuries in basketball than in football and almost the same number in baseball as in football [3].

In a systematic review and meta-analysis of mouthguard use and dental trauma, Fernandes et al. [2] found an association between use of mouthguard and prevention of dental trauma. In two different meta-analyses, athletes who wore a mouthguard were 82% and 93% less likely to suffer injury compared to those not wearing a mouthguard. Sports requiring mouthguards include Field Hockey, Football, Ice Hockey, men's and women's Lacrosse, and Wrestling if wearing orthodontic appliances. However, in a National Surveillance Study of High School Sports-Related Injuries, Collins et al. [3] found that in 72% of the traumatic dental injuries reported, no mouthguard was worn.

It is not clear why athletes don't comply with the use of equipment that has clear, compelling evidence that it prevents injury to the teeth and mouth. Possible reasons include that the athlete doesn't have a good fitting mouthguard, there is a lack of understanding of the risk for injury, the coach does not enforce the use of the mouthguard, or injury prevention is not considered to be a high priority. Parker et al. [4] summarized the barriers to mouthguard use as the following:

- Increased cost and time for fabrication of custom mouthguards
- Poorly fitting mouth formed mouthguards
- Interference with speaking and breathing
- Poor retention
- Nausea
- Negative effect on the athlete's image

Some of these barriers are clearly related to the use of poorly fitting non-custom mouthguards. The concern about "image" suggests that popular, well-known athletes may serve as role models for injury prevention behaviors such as mouthguard use.

Kroon et al., in a survey of rugby players, reported that cost and the belief that they did not work were the main reasons for not wearing a mouthguard [5]. The players also had a poor understanding of how an avulsed tooth should be managed. Spinas et al. designed a study to determine if a motivational intervention would be effective in getting basketball players to wear a mouthguard. After 12 months, 76% of the athletes who received constant motivation from coaches continued to wear a mouthguard while in the control group, only 20% continued wearing the mouthguard [6]. This suggests that enforcement from a coach or trainer is an effective method to achieve compliance with mouthguard use.

In a study of dental injuries among athletes who participate in a variety of sports, Biagi et al. found that although 80.5% of the athletes knew about the effectiveness of mouthguards for injury prevention, only 5% actually used them [7]. Finally, in studies of both college football officials and coaches, Ranalli and Lancaster reported that the majority of officials think compliance is important and that coaches should be held more accountable for the player's compliance. When coaches were surveyed, they agreed that coaches as well as players and trainers should be accountable for enforcing mouthguard use [8, 9].

Dentists play an important role in educating patients and families about the effectiveness of mouthguards to prevent dental injuries. They are also responsible for fabricating custom mouthguards for their patients. In some parts of the U.S., local dental societies have annual events where they donate their time and materials to fabricate mouthguards for high school athletes. This is a great way to bring awareness to this important safety issue and to provide mouthguards to student athletes who may not have the financial resources to do this.

There has been suggestion in the past that mouthguard use can reduce the risk of concussion injuries. This has not been shown to be true in a number of studies [10].

Helmets are recommended for many contact sports and have been shown to reduce injuries to the head and face, depending on the design. It should be noted that there are no helmets that prevent concussions [11].

10.2.1 Mouthguard Types and Fabrication

For children and adolescents who participate in sporting activities, a properly fitting athletic mouthguard is one of the most effective ways to prevent dental injuries. When used in contact sports, mouthguards have been shown to reduce dental injuries by 90% [12]. In a recent position statement by the National Athletic Trainers' Association, it was reported that orofacial injury rates in non-mouthguard mandated sports ranged from 3 to 35% and that the financial burden for a dental injury may be as high as $15,000 over the individual's lifetime [13]. For adolescents who suffer an avulsion of a permanent tooth, there are multiple trips to the dentist, root canal treatment, fabrication of a partial denture if the original treatment fails, and eventual permanent replacement of a tooth or teeth with a bridge or implant.

There are few prospective studies comparing dental injuries in athletes who wear mouthguards to those who don't. In one study, athletes were examined and fitted for custom mouthguards and then instructed in their use. After the season was complete, athletes were questioned about mouthguard use and dental injuries. There were significantly more fractured teeth in the non-mouthguard wearers compared to the mouthguard wearers [14].

One of the potential challenges related to mouthguards is the expense. A custom mouthguard fabricated by a dentist after making an impression of the patient's upper arch may cost between $60 and $500 and requires two visits to the dentist. For children in the mixed dentition, since the primary teeth are exfoliating and permanent teeth are erupting, the mouthguard is only likely to fit for one season and a new one will need to be fabricated the following year. Most dental insurance companies do not reimburse for the cost of a custom mouthguard. There are other types of mouthguards that are less expensive and don't fit as well. However, they do have some benefit and are better than using no protection. The different types of mouthguards are discussed below along with the pros and cons.

There are currently four different types of mouthguards: stock mouthguards, boil and bite (mouth formed), vacuum formed and pressure formed laminate mouthguard. Stock mouthguards are available in sporting goods stores or online, are inexpensive ($12–$20) and come in different sizes and colors. This type of mouthguard fits loosely and provides minimal protection. Athletes who wear this type of mouthguard report that it is difficult to speak or breathe when wearing them [15].

Boil and bite or mouth formed mouthguards are also available online or in sporting goods stores. They are generally made of a thermoplastic material that softens when heated in water. This type of mouthguard fits a little better than the stock mouthguards and is also inexpensive ($10–$25). Boil and bite mouthguards come in different sizes and colors and the ability to speak and breath is slightly improved compared to the stock mouthguards.

The American Dental Association recently awarded the Seal of Acceptance to one type of mouth formed mouthguard (Fig. 10.1). The Seal of Acceptance is

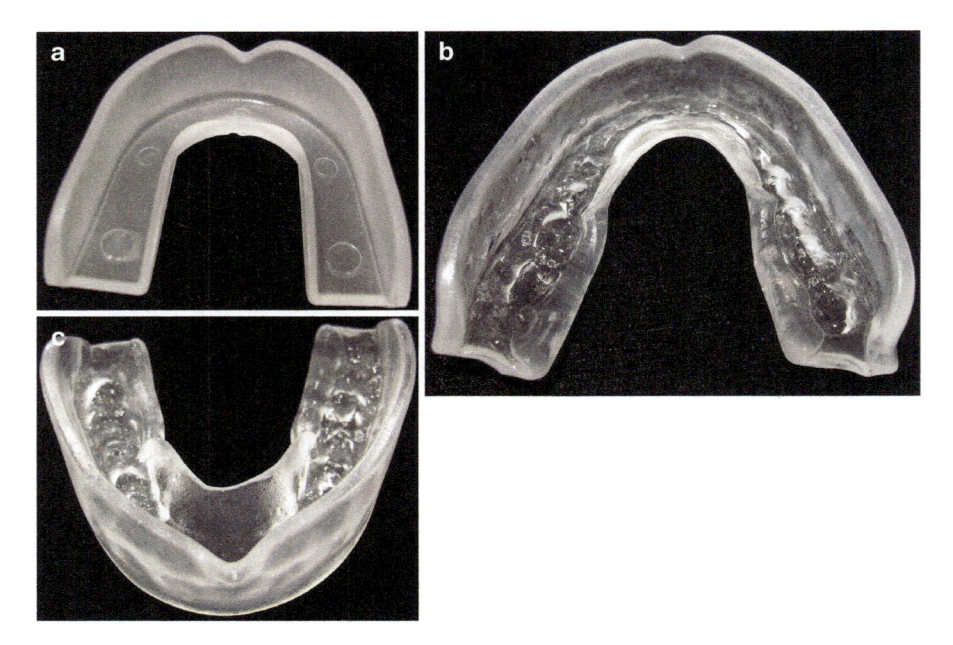

Fig. 10.1 Mouth formed mouthguard made from Vistamaxx® (Game On) as it comes out of the box (**a**). To form the mouthguard to the teeth, it is heated in the microwave, cooled briefly in ice water and then placed in mouth. The mouthguard is formed to the arch through pressure from the lips, cheeks, and tongue (**b, c**)

awarded when a product meets the safety and efficacy criteria for which the product is intended. This particular mouthguard uses a relatively new material called Vistamaxx™. Vistamaxx™ was developed by ExonMobile Chemical and is a semi-crystalline all-polyolefin propylene ethylene copolymer (PEC). In an in vitro study by Grewal and colleagues comparing custom fit laminated mouthguards with polyolefin self-adapting mouthguards, the authors concluded that the shock absorption ability of the two mouthguard materials was comparable [16]. They suggested that the polyolefin self-adapting mouthguard is an acceptable alternative to the laboratory fabricated custom mouthguard [16]. The other characteristics of polyolefin that make it appealing for use as a mouthguard are softness, flexibility, toughness, and durability [16]. One of the challenges with boil and bite mouthguards made of ethylene vinyl acetate (EVA) copolymer is the very short working time once the material is cool enough to put in the mouth. This is not an issue when this material is used to fabricate a mouthguard in the laboratory. The polyolefin materials have a wider time-temperature softness (TTS) window, allowing more time for the mouthguard to be adapted to the teeth [16].

Vacuum formed mouthguards are one type of custom mouthguard. The fabrication of this type of mouthguard requires making an impression of the child's teeth (usually the upper arch), creating a stone model of the teeth and then using a specialized device to heat the sheet of mouthguard material and form it onto the stone model using a vacuum suction machine. This type of mouthguard fits snugly onto the teeth, does not interfere with speaking and breathing, and is considered the industry standard. The cost is more than the stock or boil and bite mouthguards and may range from $200 to $500.

Pressure formed laminate mouthguards are a second type of custom mouthguard (Fig. 10.2a, b). The process of making this type of mouthguard is similar to that described for the vacuum formed type in terms of the impression and stone model creation. A vacuum suction machine is used that makes it possible to use multiple

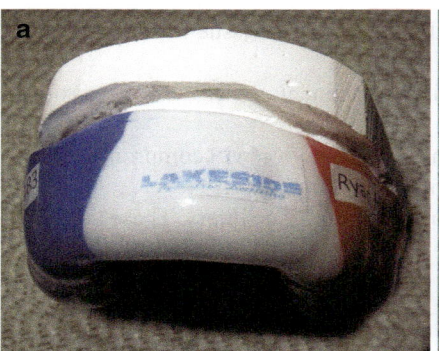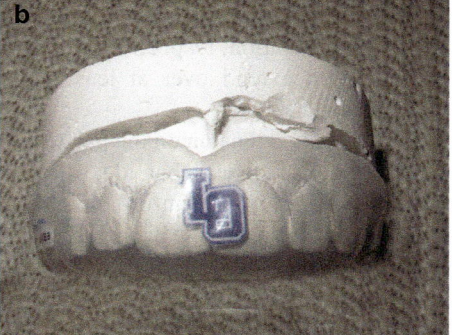

Fig. 10.2 Pressure formed laminate mouthguards (**a, b**). These are considered custom mouthguards and are made by making an impression of the maxillary arch, creating a stone model and then using a vacuum suction machine to heat and adapt the material to the model. (Courtesy of Dr. Ryan Hughes)

layers of material. The machine used for this type of mouthguard is a positive pressure machine. Examples include Erkopress-2004, Biostar, and Druformat. In these machines, after the mouthguard material is heated, it is pressed onto the stone model with negative pressure from below. This improves the adaptation to the cast and facilitates creation of a thicker, laminated mouthguard. It is preferable to limit the thickness to 4 mm to ensure both protection and comfort for the wearer [17].

For both types of custom mouthguards, it is important to follow the recommended steps to ensure the best fitting, most protective appliance [17]. These steps are outlined below:

1. Make an alginate impression of the maxillary arch including all teeth and with extension into the vestibule.
2. Make a stone cast from the impression and allow it to dry thoroughly before making the mouthguard.
3. Trim the stone model so that the vestibule is mostly removed.
4. Drill a hole in the palatal portion of the cast (about the size of a dime). This will improve the suction and adaptation of the EVA plate to the cast.
5. Heat the EVA plate (mouthguard material) until it droops down toward the cast about 2–2.5 cm (3/4–1 in).
6. Engage the vacuum machine to form the mouthguard material over the cast.
7. Allow the material to cool completely before removing it from the cast.
8. Carefully trim the mouthguard so that it extends into the vestibule, at least up to the second molar and is relieved in the area of the buccal and labial frena.
9. The cut edges should be smoothed with a flame or a rag-wheel.
10. Any areas that are impinging on tissues can be further trimmed at the time the patient tries it in.

Sigurdsson and Cohenca [17] discuss a number of common errors that may occur when fabricating custom mouthguards. These include:

1. Over or under extension of the material will cause soft tissue irritation or compromise retention, respectively.
2. Failure to extend over at least the first permanent molar will compromise retention.
3. Insufficient extension on the palate in the anterior region will compromise retention and provide less than ideal strength for the mouthguard.
4. Rough edges are uncomfortable and can cause soft tissue injury. These are easily smoothed with a flame or rag-wheel.

10.3 Bicycle: Helmets

Accidents involving riding bicycles are relatively common and result in injuries to the head, limbs, and teeth. Twenty-two U.S. states require children to wear a bicycle helmet [18]. The age requirement varies by state and it is unclear how frequently these laws are enforced. Internationally, a number of countries have mandatory helmet laws either for all ages or just for children.

When worn properly, helmets protect against head injuries but may or may not protect against facial or dental injuries. A recent policy statement from the American Academy of Pediatrics [19] states that 88% of serious brain injuries can be prevented by the use of bicycle helmets. Bicycle helmets have been shown to reduce both the number and severity of head injuries [20]. In addition, helmets have been shown to reduce the severity of upper and midface injuries but not lower face injuries [21]. Since the maxillary incisors are the teeth most frequently injured during falls, the use of a bicycle helmet should be encouraged to prevent both head injuries and dental injuries.

Amadori et al. 2017 reported on bicycle injuries in Italian children. Medical records from 1405 patients were assessed. The most common age for injury in this group was in children between 8 and 10 years old. Fractures of teeth were the most common injury. Ninety percent of the teeth injured were permanent teeth. The most common teeth to be injured were maxillary central incisors. Maxillofacial fractures occurred in 11% of patients. Only 3% of the cases wore a protective helmet [22].

Caregivers are primarily responsible for enforcing the use of bicycle helmets and are important role models for their children and adolescents. Caregivers use of a helmet when accompanying their child on a bike ride and mandatory state helmet laws have both been strongly associated with helmet use by children [23]. However, dentists, physicians, and other health care providers should also provide regular education and anticipatory guidance regarding the importance of this preventive equipment. These health care professionals also play an important role in advocating for changes in state laws to promote bicycle helmet use.

10.4 Excessive Overjet

Protrusive maxillary incisors have been shown to put a child at increased risk for dental trauma. The greater the degree of overjet, the greater the risk of trauma [24]. When excess overjet is diagnosed, it is an opportunity to educate families about the increased risk for dental trauma and to discuss options to decrease risk. This includes orthodontic correction of the overjet and/or protective equipment such as athletic mouthguard, helmet, or facemask, depending on the activity the child is involved in.

10.5 Attention-Deficit Hyperactivity Disorder (ADHD)

According to the Attention-Deficit/Hyperactivity Disorder (ADHD) Institute [25], the prevalence worldwide of this disorder for children and adolescents is between 5.3 and 7.1% making it one of the most common neurodevelopmental disorders of childhood. It affects individuals of all ages and has been reported to have a higher prevalence among males. The primary characteristics of ADHD are hyperactivity, inattentiveness, and impulsivity. In addition, their increased accident proneness contributes to the risk for injury of all types, including dental [26].

It has been recognized for over 10 years that children and adolescents with ADHD are at increased risk for traumatic dental injuries. In a recent review of the literature, 9 out of 12 studies confirmed the link between ADHD and TDI in children and adolescents [27]. The increased risk for dental trauma among children with ADHD is estimated to be three times that of children without ADHD [28].

The prevention of dental traumatic injuries in children with ADHD may be more challenging than for children without this disorder because of their impulsivity and accident proneness. However, there is evidence in the medical literature that pharmacologic treatment of ADHD is effective in managing a child's behavior and decreases their risk for traumatic injuries [29].

10.6   Automobile Injuries

Seat belts, car seats, and airbags have significantly decreased the number and severity of injuries related to automobile accidents. In the United States, the National Highway Traffic Safety Administration estimated that the use of seatbelts and airbags was 75% effective in preventing serious head injuries [30]. More recent data showed that seat belt use increased from 82.5% in 2007 to 90.1% in 2016 [30].

The incidence and severity of maxillofacial injuries occurred in 1 out of 449 accidents when the driver and passenger used both seat belts and airbags while this rate was 1 in 40 for individuals that used neither seat belts or airbags [31]. Many states have laws regarding the use of child restraints such as car seats and booster seats. The lowest risk of injury occurs when age appropriate safety restraints are used in the rear seat of the car. Inappropriately restrained children were at almost twice the risk of injury and unrestrained children were at greater than three times the risk of injury [32]. A study focusing on the etiology of mandibular fractures reported that the most common cause of mandibular fracture was from road traffic accidents (68%) and the second most common was fall from a height (30%) [33]. In this study, the male to female ratio was 4.5:1.

10.7   Violence

Child abuse/maltreatment is a global issue and effects children of all ages, races, and nationalities. Physical abuse is one component of child abuse with more than half of the injuries involving the head, neck, and face [34]. When the description of an injury doesn't match what is seen clinically, there should be further investigation. For example, preambulatory children rarely have bruises and bruises to the torso, ears, and neck in children under 4 are suggestive of abuse [35].

Fighting has been documented as one of the causes of dental trauma in adolescents. Maxillofacial trauma as a result of interpersonal violence (IPV) has been reported to have a prevalence rate ranging from 9 to 52% [36]. In a study of 790 patients with maxillofacial trauma from IPV, 17% were found to have dental trauma.

These numbers included both domestic and urban violence. Four percent of those with dental trauma were under 19 years of age [36].

In a study of 6000 patients (of all ages) with facial injuries, 48% had dental trauma. Of those with dental trauma, 36% were from acts of violence [37].

One of the challenges of gathering reliable data about the prevalence of maxillofacial and dental trauma is that there is not a central repository for this information. For injuries that are primarily dental in nature, the patient is most likely seen by their dentist of record. If the injury is more extensive or involves the face, jaws, or head, the patient is more likely to be seen in a hospital emergency room and managed by a maxillofacial surgeon. National trauma databases exist in a number of countries and generally collect data for traumatic injuries requiring a visit to the emergency room or hospitalization. Some of these databases include maxillofacial injuries [38, 39] but none include dental injuries.

INSPIRE is a collaboration between the World Health Organization and multiple US and international agencies including the United States Centers for Disease Control and Prevention (CDC), End Violence Against Children: The Global Partnership, the Pan American Health Organization (PAHO), the President's Emergency Program for AIDS Relief (PEPFAR), Together for Girls, the United Nations Children's Fund (UNICEF), United Nations Office on Drugs and Crime (UNODC), United States Agency for International Development (USAID), and the World Bank. INSPIRE is an acronym for the seven strategies for ending violence against children: Implementation and enforcement of laws; Norms and values; Safe environments; Parent and caregiver support; Income and economic strengthening; Response and support services; and Education and life skills [40]. In the document describing these strategies, the authors cite survey data on the prevalence of violence against children in 96 countries which estimates that one billion children globally—over half of all children aged 2–17 years—have experienced emotional, physical, or sexual violence in the past year. Physical violence resulting in traumatic dental injuries is included in these numbers and presumably, strategies to end violence against children would be effective for that subset of injuries that result in dental trauma.

Violence against children is multidimensional and efforts to prevent it must be focused on multiple areas simultaneously [40]. The areas that apply to physical violence resulting in traumatic dental injuries include:

(a) Identifying families at risk for violence and providing support to create a nurturing environment
(b) Physical changes of unsafe environments
(c) Reduce the risk of violence in public spaces where children and adolescents gather
(d) Change cultural attitudes that foster violence
(e) Limit access to harmful agents such as guns and alcohol
(f) Ensure good quality response service for children affected by violence
(g) Eliminate the cultural, social, and economic inequalities that contribute to violence

10.8 Summary

Most of the evidence about traumatic dental injuries confirms that there is still a significant amount of education that needs to be provided to patients, families, coaches, trainers, teachers, and health care providers. Anyone who interacts with children in a home, school, or sports setting should know how to prevent injury and what to do if a dental injury occurs, especially permanent tooth avulsion.

How traumatic dental injuries are managed has a dramatic influence on the long-term survival of the tooth. Being familiar with the IADT guidelines and having the necessary materials and expertise to follow these guidelines is crucial. It is impossible to predict when a child with a traumatic dental injury will present to the office so being prepared for a traumatic dental injury is very similar to being prepared for any other type of emergency. Having a Trauma Kit easily available will decrease the stress of the dental team and the patient and increase the likelihood of a positive outcome.

References

1. American Academy of Pediatric Dentistry. Periodicity of examination, preventive dental services, anticipatory guidance/counseling, and oral treatment for infants, children, and adolescents. AAPD Reference Manual, Vol. 40; 2018. p. 194–203. http://www.aapd.org/media/Policies_Guidelines/BP_Periodicity.pdf. Accessed 5/11/2019.
2. Fernandes LM, Neto JCL, Lima TFR, Magno MB, Santiago BM, Cavalcanti YW, de Almeida LFD. The use of mouthguards and prevalence of dento-alveolar trauma among athletes: a systematic review and meta-analysis. Dent Traumatol. 2018;. https://onlinelibrary.wiley.com/doi/epdf/10.1111/edt.12441
3. Collins CL, McKenzie LB, Ferketich RA, Huiyun X, Comstock RD. Dental injuries sustained by high school athletes in the United States, from 2008/2009 through 2013/2014 academic years. Dent Traumatol. 2016;32:121–7.
4. Parker K, Marlow B, Patel N, Gill DS. A review of mouthguards: effectiveness, types, characteristics and indications for use. Br Dent J. 2017;222:629–33.
5. Kroon J, Cox JA, Knight JE, Nevins PN, Kong WW. Mouthguard use and awareness of junior rugby league players in the gold coast, Australia: a need for more education. Clin J Sport Med. 2016;26:128–32.
6. Spinas E, Aresu M, Giannetti L. Use of mouth guard in basketball: observational study of a group of teenagers with and without motivational reinforcement. Eur J Paediatr Dent. 2014;15:392–6.
7. Biagi R, Cardarelli F, Butti AC, Salvato A. Sports-related dental injuries: knowledge of first aid and mouthguard use in a sample of Italian children and youngsters. Eur J Paediatr Dent. 2010;11:66–70.
8. Ranalli DN, Lancaster DM. Attitudes of college football officials regarding NCAA mouthguard regulations and player compliance. J Public Health Dent. 1993;53:96–00.
9. Ranalli DN, Lancaster DM. Attitudes of college football coaches regarding NCAA mouthguard regulations and player compliance. J Public Health Dent. 1995;55:139–42.
10. Lloyd JD, Nakamura WS, Maeda Y, Takeda T, Leesungbok R, Lazarchik D, Dorney B, Gonda T, Nakajima K, Yasui T, Iwata Y, Suzuki H, Tsukimura N, Churei H, Kwon KR, Choy MMH, Rock JB. Mouthguards and their use in sports: Report of the 1st International Sports Dentistry Workshop. Dent Traumatol. 2017;33:421–6.

11. Centers for Disease Control and Prevention. Child safety and injury prevention. Safe Child. www.cdc.gov/safechild/. Accessed 1/7/19.

12. Chapman PJ, Nasser BP. Prevalence of orofacial injuries and use of mouthguards in high school Rugby Union. Aust Dent J. 1996;41:252–5.

13. Gould TE, Piland SG, Caswell SV, Ranalli D, Mills S, Ferrara MS, Courson R. National Athletic Trainers' Association Position Statement: preventing and managing sport-related dental and oral injuries. J Athl Train. 2016;51:821–39.

14. Morton JG, Burton JF. An evaluation of the effectiveness of mouthguards in high-school rugby players. N Z Dent J. 1979;75:151–3.

15. Duddy FA, Weissman J, Lee RA Sr, Paranjpe A, Johnson JD, Cohenca N. Influence of different types of mouthguards on strength and performance of collegiate athletes: a controlled-randomized trial. Dent Traumatol. 2012;28:263–7.

16. Grewal N, Kumari F, Tiwari U. Comparative evaluation of shock absorption ability of custom-fit mouthguards with new-generation polyolefin self-adapting mouthguards in three different maxillary anterior teeth alignments using Fiber Bragg Grating (FBG) sensors. Dent Traumatol. 2015;31:294–01.

17. Sigurdsson A, Cohenca N. Prevention of dental and oral injuries. In: Andreasen JO, Andreasen FM, Andersson L, editors. Textbook and color atlas of traumatic injuries to the teeth. 5th ed. Hoboken: Wiley-Blackwell; 2019. p. 933–54.

18. Bicycle Helmet Safety Institute. https://www.helmets.org/mandator.htm#international. Accessed 1/7/19.

19. American Academy of Pediatrics. Committee on Injury and Poison Prevention. Pediatrics. 2001;108:1030–2.

20. Chapman HR, Curran AL. Bicycle helmets—does the dental profession have a role in promoting their use? Br Dent J. 2004;196:555–60.

21. Thompson DC, Nunn ME, Thompson RS, Rivara F. Effectiveness of bicycle safety helmets in preventing serious facial injury. JAMA. 1996;276:1974–5.

22. Amadori F, Bardellini E, Copeta A, Conti G, Villa V, Majorana A. Dental trauma and bicycle safety: a report in Italian children and adolescents. Acta Odontol Scand. 2017;75:227–31.

23. Parkin PC, Spence LJ, Hu X, Kranz KE, Shortt LG, Wesson DE. Evaluation of a promotional strategy to increase bicycle helmet use by children. Pediatrics. 1993;91:772–7.

24. Petti S. Over two hundred million injuries to anterior teeth attributable to large overjet: a meta-analysis. Dent Traumatol. 2015;31:1–8.

25. Attention Deficit Hyperactivity Disorder Institute. https://adhd-institute.com/burden-of-adhd/epidemiology/. Accessed 1/7/19.

26. Sabuncuoglu O, Taser H, Berkem M. Relationship between traumatic dental injuries and attention-deficit/hyperactivity disorder in children and adolescents: proposal of an explanatory model. Dent Traumatol. 2005;21:249–53.

27. Sabuncuoglu O, Irmak MY. The attention-deficit/hyperactivity disorder model for traumatic dental injuries: a critical review and update of the last 10 years. Dent Traumatol. 2017;33:71–6.

28. Ziegler AM. Analysis of a comprehensive dental trauma database: an epidemiologic study of traumatic dental injuries to the permanent dentition. Dissertation, The Ohio State University; 2014.

29. Man KK, Chan EW, Coghill D, Douglas I, Ip P, Leung LP, Tsui MS, Wong WH, Wong IC. Methylphenidate and the risk of trauma. Pediatrics. 2015;135:40–8.

30. Traffic safety facts 1997. National Highway Traffic Safety Administration, US Dept of Transportation. Publication DOT HS 808770; 1998.

31. Mouzakes J, Koltai PJ, Kuhar S, Bernstein DS, Wing P, Salsberg E. The impact of airbags and seat belts on the incidence and severity of maxillofacial injuries in automobile accidents in New York State. Arch Otolaryngol Head Neck Surg. 2001;127:1189–93.

32. Durbin DR, Chen I, Smith R, Elliott MR, Winston FK. Effects of seating position and appropriate restraint use on the risk of injury to children in motor vehicle crashes. Pediatrics. 2005;115:e305–9.

33. Natu SS, Pradhan H, Gupta H, Alam S, Gupta S, Pradhan R, Mohammad S, Kohli M, Sinha VP Shankar R, Agarwal A. An epidemiological study on pattern and incidence of mandibular fractures. Plast Surg Int. 2012;2012:834364.
34. Fisher-Owens SA, Lukefahr JL, Tate AR, American Academy of Pediatrics, Section on Oral Health, Committee on Child Abuse and Neglect, American Academy of Pediatric Dentistry, Council on Clinical affairs, Council on Scientific Affairs, Ad Hoc Work Group on Child Abuse and Neglect. Oral and dental aspects of child abuse and neglect. Pediatr Dent. 2017;39:278–83.
35. Christian CW, Committee on Child Abuse and Neglect, American Academy of Pediatrics. The evaluation of suspected child physical abuse. Pediatrics. 2015;135:e1337–54.
36. Ferreira MC, Batista AM, Ferreira FO, Ramos-Joege ML, Marques LS. Pattern of oral-maxillofacial trauma stemming from interpersonal physical violence and determinant factors. Dent Traumatol. 2014;30:15–21.
37. Gassner R, Bosch R, Tuli T, Emshoff R. Prevalence of dental trauma in 6000 patients with facial injuries: implications for prevention. Oral Surg Oral Med Oral Pathol Oral Radiol Endod. 1999;87(1):27–33.
38. Levin L, Lin S, Goldman S, Peleg K. Relationship between socio-economic position and general, maxillofacial and dental trauma: A National Trauma Registry Study. Dent Traumatol. 2010;26:342–5.
39. American College of Surgeons National Trauma Data Bank Pediatric report. 2016. https://www.facs.org/quality-programs/trauma/tqp/center-programs/ntdb/docpub. Accessed 12/7/18.
40. World Health Organization. INSPIRE: seven strategies for ending violence against children. 2016. https://www.who.int/violence_injury_prevention/violence/inspire/en/. Accessed 12/28/18.